Better Mental Health Care

Better Mental Health Care

By

Graham Thornicroft

Professor of Community Psychiatry
Head of Health Service and Population Research Department
Institute of Psychiatry
King's College London
London, UK

and

Michele Tansella

Professor of Psychiatry
Department of Medicine and Public Health
Section of Psychiatry and Clinical Psychology
University of Verona
Verona, Italy

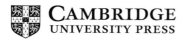
CAMBRIDGE
UNIVERSITY PRESS

CAMBRIDGE UNIVERSITY PRESS
Cambridge, New York, Melbourne, Madrid, Cape Town, Singapore, São Paulo, Delhi

Cambridge University Press
The Edinburgh Building, Cambridge CB2 8RU, UK

Published in the United States of America by Cambridge University Press, New York

www.cambridge.org
Information on this title: www.cambridge.org/9780521689465

First published 2009

Printed in the United Kingdom at the University Press, Cambridge

A catalogue record for this publication is available from the British Library

Library of Congress Cataloguing in Publication data
Thornicroft, Graham.
Better mental health care / by Graham Thornicroft and Michele Tansella.
    p.   ;   cm.
Includes index.
ISBN 978-0-521-68946-5 (pbk.)
1. Mental health services.   I. Tansella, Michele.   II. Title.
[DNLM: 1. Mental Health Services.   2. Evidence-Based Medicine.   3. Mental Disorders.
4. Outcome and Process Assessment (Health Care) – methods. WM 30 T512b   2009]
RA790.T515   2009
362.2–dc22

                                                                        2008036967

ISBN 978-0-521-68946-5 paperback

Contents

Foreword

By Dr. Benedetto Saraceno, Director, Department of Mental Health and Substance Abuse, World Health Organization, Geneva, Switzerland.

This book by Graham Thornicroft and Michele Tansella has a very clear objective: how better care could achieve better outcomes for people suffering from mental disorders. The preoccupation of the book is to derive better mental health care from the best ethical, evidence-based and experience-based practices available. These two propositions, improving outcomes and framing interventions upon ethics, evidence and experience, are so clearly defined by the authors that this book represents a challenge to psychiatrists who sometimes forget the key link between 'treatment' and 'care'. I say this because I was surprised to note, when looking at the themes of the World Congress of Psychiatry 2008, that among the most disparate issues in the list the words: policy; plan; service; are not even mentioned.

This book talks about community care and, overcoming the numerous theoretical debates around this issue, simply states that community care means services close to home and that a modern mental health service is a balance between community-based and hospital-based care. The authors stress that the evidence available, but also the experience accumulated, support an approach where the provision of hospital care is limited, while the most important part of the care should be delivered at community level. The debate about the balance between hospital and community care (whether the former should prevail over the latter or vice versa) has lasted for many years, and this book provides a solid answer, after which it would be difficult for the debate to continue as ethical, evidence-based and experience-based elements support the idea of a balanced approach which includes community care with a limited provision of hospital care. The authors discuss the resources needed to establish new services outside hospitals and this, too, is an old debate; in some cases the lack of resources argument has been used to justify the perpetuation of an exclusively hospital-based model.

What clearly emerges from the book is that while extra resources are very difficult to identify, the transfer of resources from hospital to community services is a realistic and viable model. This is an important point because it shows that service planners cannot build a parallel service, community and hospital, without clearly decreasing the investment in hospitals, liberating resources and moving those resources towards community services.

Of course, moving care from hospitals, which are, by definition, the health professionals' fiefdom, to the community, where the power of service-users is more embedded in the day-to-day care delivery than in a hospital setting, raises another important issue, which is the one of service-users' involvement. Again the book is clear about this. Service-users should be partners in care, which means that treatment plans are negotiated between health-providers and service-users. In addition, family members should be involved. In other words, the community service involvement becomes a dynamic, interactive setting where negotiation becomes a key word which confirms the initial statement of the book, namely that ethics, experience and science should go hand in hand. Care based on ethics and experience without science is not good, but, equally, care based on experience and science without ethics is unacceptable. In this sense the book by Thornicroft and Tansella brings fresh air into the present debate about mental health care and service organisation.

It is also interesting that the book raises the issue of different resource settings, which is quite uncommon and very much appreciated by someone like me, from the World Health Organization. In fact, the book talks about low-, medium- and high-income countries in relation to the type of service provision they can offer. The low-income countries can often only rely upon primary health care with very scarce specialist back-up, while middle-income countries can provide outpatient ambulatory clinics, community mental health teams, acute in-patient care, long-term community-based residential care and, finally, rehabilitation and work. Here, the authors have two very interesting messages. The first is the emphasis on rehabilitation and its role within mental health services. The second is that the authors, when talking about long-term residential care, refer to community-based residential care, which means that in their minds long-term residential care cannot be synonymous with traditional psychiatric hospitals.

This attention to low- and middle-income countries is important and also makes the book a valuable instrument for those health professionals, care providers and planners who work in less resourced settings. The authors recognise that to achieve this kind of balanced approach and to reach a high-quality mental health community service there are a number of barriers that should be recognised and challenged. The authors echo some elements from the Lancet Series on Global Mental Health and specifically from *Barriers to Improvement of Mental Health Services in Low-Income and Middle-Income Countries*, Saraceno *et al.* The authors recognise that insufficient funding, centralization of resources, large institutions, complexities in mainstreaming mental health care in primary health care, scarcity of health workers trained in mental health, poor public health vision among mental-health leaders and fragmentation, if not sometimes contradiction between mental health advocacy groups, are the key barriers to be overcome.

However, other barriers described by Thornicroft and Tansella are playing a role in making the change difficult. The authors stress that the research evidence in mental health is mainly concentrated at an individual level rather than at a local level and that the evidence generally applies to single clinical interventions rather than to treatment combinations, such as medication plus psychological support plus psychosocial rehabilitation. In other words, the authors think that the clinical approach still prevails in research, not a more service-oriented approach. Accordingly, research should be more service oriented because service organisations clearly play a role in outcome determination. Patients do not improve or worsen just because they received one medication or another, but because this treatment was provided in a certain care environment or another. Therefore, treatment cannot be seen in a vacuum, but occurs in the framework of a service organisation and the characteristics of each service organisation are powerful determinants of the evolution of a disorder and the outcome of its treatment.

What clearly emerges from this compelling book is that moving services from institutions to the community does not require, in the authors' words, 'purely a physical relocation of treatment sites, but requires a fundamental reorientation of staff attitudes'.

Finally, in their delightful intermezzo on the history of mental health care, the authors mention three historical periods:

(1) The rise of the asylum
(2) The decline of the asylum
(3) The development of centralised community-based mental health care.

The authors' assumption would appear to be that we are living in the third period, which I think optimistic. Undoubtedly the services they lead in their respective countries, the UK and Italy, belong to the third period, but the majority of services, even in some economically developed nations, are still in period two, the decline of the asylum, not having yet reached period three. There are also signs in some countries that history is reversing to the first period and a new type of asylum could appear, possibly with different external characteristics from those sad images with which we are familiar when looking back to the reality of large asylums; nevertheless there are new types of asylum growing and, in some countries, this is represented by prisons. A large number of people suffering from mental disorders now live in prisons and these institutions are characterised by the same logic of the old psychiatric asylums and are very far from the idea of a decentralised, community-based mental health service. A further example is institutions for the elderly, which are not technically defined as psychiatric asylums, but they are long-term institutions for people with mental disorders such as dementia.

On this slightly pessimistic note, I wish to congratulate Professor Thornicroft and Professor Tansella for once again contributing to better mental health care with a book that will help policy-makers, service-planners, mental health professionals, family and consumer organisations and, also, on behalf of the World Health Organization, I wish to thank them for this remarkable contribution.

Acknowledgements

We wish to acknowledge the many people who have encouraged us and who have directly helped us with this book. In particular we would like to thank: Abdul Aziz Abdullah, Thomas Becker, Chee Kok Yoon, Fiona Crowley, Cecília Cruz Villares, Nicolas Daumerie, Iris De Coster, Melvyn Freeman, Nikos Gionakis, Peykan G. Gökalp, Sergiu Grozavu, Lars Hansson, Judit Harangozo, Ulrich Junghan, Yiannis Kalakoutas, Alisher Latypov, Burul Makenbaeva, Graham Mellsop, Roberto Mezzina, Pĕtr Nawka, Jean Luc Roelandt, Vesna Švab, Maris Taube, Radu Teodorescu, Rita Thom, Chantal Van Audenhove, Jaap van Weeghel, Kristian Wahlbeck, Richard Warner and Stefan Weinmann, who have directly engaged with us on the questions and challenges discussed in Chapter 6. Dr. Ann Law also provided invaluable contributions, both to Chapter 6 and to the volume as a whole. Richard Marley at Cambridge University Press has been a source of continuous support throughout this project. We have also developed the approach described here through informal discussions, in many parts of the world, with people active across the whole range of mental health care, who have offered us ideas and inspiration: some who plan services, others who provide care, and the many who need better mental health care.

Beginning the journey: mapping the route

Aim of the book: how to improve mental health care

The reform of mental health services is now proceeding in many countries throughout the world. Although the speed and the local details of these changes vary between countries, there is a clear need for an overall map, which can assist all those service-users, family members and staff involved in this transformation. In a sense this book acts as a guide, providing a compass to orientate the direction of travel.

The mental health care changes we shall discuss are reforms in two senses. On one hand they are a profound re-orientation of the principles which guide how treatment and care should be provided to people with mental illness. On the other hand they also refer to changes in the physical shape and pattern of health- and social-care services. In this book we shall provide a practical manual to help people who are involved in improving mental health services, and offering guidance in relation to three key cornerstones: the ethical foundation, the evidence base and the accumulation of experience which has been gathered in recent years.

First, the ethical foundation refers to establishing agreed fundamental principles which orientate how service planning, provision and evaluation should be conducted. For example, is it more important to emphasise continuity of care in a service, or to focus upon accessibility, or should both be local priorities? Second we shall highlight the importance of providing, wherever possible, interventions and services which are soundly evidence-based, for example those shown to be effective in routine clinical settings in systematic reviews, based on the results of randomised controlled trials. Third, we shall also draw upon a range of other types of evidence, such as knowledge stemming from the experience accrued from good clinical practice, especially in those areas of clinical practice which have not yet been subjected to formal evaluation. In our view the foremost of these guideposts is the ethical base, as this provides the foundation stone for deciding what types of evidence and experience should be valued most highly [1].

Table 1.1 The Matrix Model

Place Dimension	Time Dimension		
	(A) Input Phase	(B) Process Phase	(C) Outcome Phase
(1) Country /Regional Level	1A	1B	1C
(2) Local Level	2A	2B	2C
(3) Individual Level	3A	3B	3C

A clear limitation of this book is that it focuses upon our own experience in Western Europe, and so includes less information from other continents [2;3]. We shall try to balance this by including illustrations by colleagues in 25 countries worldwide, in which they describe their experiences (both positive and negative) in developing mental health care, so the lessons they have learned can also assist you.

Drawing the map: the 'matrix model'

We believe that a map is necessary to help shape service aims and the steps necessary for their implementation. To be useful such a map should be simple. We have therefore created a scheme with only two dimensions, which we call the *matrix model.*

Our aim is that this model will help you to assess the relative strengths and weaknesses of local services, and to formulate a clear plan of action to improve them. We also expect that the matrix model will assist you by offering a step-by-step approach that is clear, but is also flexible enough to be relevant to your local circumstances.

The two *dimensions* of this map are place and time (see Table 1.1). Place refers to three geographical levels: (1) country/regional; (2) local and (3) individual. The second dimension (time) refers to three phases: (A) inputs; (B) processes and (C) outcomes. Using these two dimensions we can make a 3×3 matrix to bring into focus critical issues for mental health care.

We have chosen to include the geographical dimension in the matrix because we believe that mental health services should be primarily organised locally, to be delivered to individuals in need. However, some of the key factors are decided regionally or nationally, for example overall financial allocations to the mental health sector. In this sense, therefore, the local level acts as a lens to focus policies and resources most effectively for the benefit of individual service-users.

We have selected time as the other organising dimension, as we see a clear sequence of events flowing from inputs to processes to outcomes. In our view outcomes should be the most important element, and the mental health system as a whole should be judged on the outcomes it produces.

One of our aims is that this matrix model can assist, in a sense, the accurate diagnosis of dysfunctional mental health services so that corrective action can be applied at the right level(s) to improve care. At the same time, this model is not intended to be rigidly prescriptive. It can be taken as a tool to use in analysing problems, and then in deciding what action to take. We encourage you to adapt these ideas to maximise their relevance to your local situation.

Illustrations of using the matrix model

The practical use of the matrix model is the central theme of this book. One illustration of this is how the model can help us to understand which factors contribute to a good outcome for a person with an acute episode of severe mental illness who is treated at home. Such an outcome is often seen as a success for the practitioners who work at the *individual level*, but, in fact, also depends upon decisions made at the *local level* (e.g. to provide home treatment services), and in addition may be enabled by policies and resources decided at the *national level* (e.g. to develop community care).

How to use the resources and ideas in this book

To make this book as useful as possible for you we shall provide an array of resources from which you can choose. The main ideas will be presented in the text, accompanied by tables and figures to show them graphically. In addition we shall offer text-boxes, which include relevant quotations, by service-users, family members and staff, of their experiences, linked to the themes of each chapter. There will also be special feature-boxes, with examples of good practice on specific topics. Throughout the text you will also find references to the background literature, with full details provided at the end of each chapter, in case you want to go back to these primary sources. We shall try to keep the book free of jargon. Each chapter will end with a summary of the key points to reinforce the main issues addressed.

Although we shall attempt to make balanced and fair use of the available research evidence, at the same time we need to say that we are not neutral. We would like to make clear to you our own bias. We have both undergone a medical training, and we now place ourselves in the traditions of epidemiological psychiatry, and public-health medicine. From these traditions we attach a very high value to an evidence-based approach. In addition, we believe, from our own experience, in the importance of a direct interplay between research and clinical practice, which should be mutually beneficial. Indeed we consider that the medical model alone (without taking into account social, psychological and economic factors) is insufficient to understand the full complexity of mental disorders, their causes and their consequences for people with these conditions and their family members.

This new book is written following our earlier volume, called *The Mental Health Matrix* [4]. Our approach remains consistent; how to offer ideas that will be practically useful to those of us who are trying to make mental health services better. Whereas the earlier book was written for a more research-orientated readership, here we intend to provide useful ideas for a wider range of people, including service-users, family members, practitioners and students of the mental health professions, and so the core ideas are presented directly in relation to examples from clinical practice. Second, we have substantially updated the evidence base, which has changed a great deal over the last decade. Third, having discussed the matrix model with many colleagues worldwide in recent years, it is clear that it should be considered as an approach which can be flexibly adopted according to local circumstances, in high-, medium- and low-resource countries. For this reason we shall include many real examples from colleagues who have tried to make changes for the better, sometimes succeeding and sometimes not.

Key points in this chapter

- The matrix model can be used as a map to guide decisions about how to improve mental health services.
- The matrix model includes two dimensions: time (inputs, processes and outcomes) and place (national, local and individual levels).
- Planning needs to consider knowledge from three domains: ethics, evidence and experience.

REFERENCES

1. Thornicroft G and Tansella M. Translating ethical principles into outcome measures for mental health service research. *Psychol. Med.* 1999; **29**(4):761–767.
2. Desjarlais R, Eisenberg L, Good B and Kleinman A. *World Mental Health. Problems and Priorities in Low Income Countries.* Oxford: Oxford University Press; 1995.
3. Ben-Tovim D. *Development Psychiatry. Mental Health and Primary Health Care in Botswana.* London: Tavistock; 1987.
4. Thornicroft G and Tansella M. *The Mental Health Matrix: A Manual to Improve Services.* Cambridge: Cambridge University Press; 1999.

2

Mental health of the population and care in the community

What does 'community' mean?

We shall discuss at the outset the key question: what is the meaning of *'community'*? Table 2.1 shows five definitions of 'community', selected from the *Concise Oxford Dictionary*. In relation to the focus of this book, the first two meanings ('all the people living in a specific locality', 'a specific locality, including its inhabitants'), are most important as they reflect our view that mental-health services are best organised for defined local areas, for *all* local residents who need treatment or care. Within any local population there are likely to be specific sub-groups who are at higher risk for mental disorders, or whose needs for services are distinct. Such groups include immigrants, people who are homeless, or those exposed to particular environmental or biological risk factors, such as disaster or bereavement.

The last two of these definitions shown in Table 2.1 also have important implications, namely when 'community' refers to the 'fellowship of interests of the general public' as a whole. This wider community of citizens in fact delegates responsibility for the care of mentally ill people to the mental health services. One aspect of this approach is that mental health staff are expected to provide a public service, not only by treating, but also by removing or containing, those who pose a risk to the public safety.

Defining 'community care' and 'community mental health'

In essence, 'community care' means services close to home. The term 'community care' was first officially used in Britain, for example, in 1957 [2;3;4], and its historical development has been interpreted in four ways to mean: (i) care outside large institutions; (ii) professional services provided outside hospitals; (iii) care by the community or (iv) normalisation in ordinary living [5]. Taking into account these roots of 'community', how can *community mental health*

Table 2.1 Definitions of 'Community'

Community
(1) All the people living in a specific locality
(2) A specific locality, including its inhabitants
(3) Body of people having a religion, a profession, etc., in common (*the immigrant community*)
(4) Fellowship of interests etc.; similarity (*community of intellect*)
(5) The public

Source: Concise Oxford Dictionary [1]

services be defined? Table 2.2 shows a selection of key definitions which have appeared over the last 35 years.

Integral to this most recent definition is our view that a modern mental health service is a balance between community-based and hospital-based care, which replaces the traditional, more custodial system dominated by large mental hospitals and out-patient clinics offering follow-up care, usually limiting treatment to medication [6].

The public health approach to mental health

What does the 'public health approach' mean? The origins of the public health approach lie in the concept of 'social medicine', which Virchow introduced into Germany in 1948 [7], proposing the reform of medicine on the basis of four principles:
(1) The health of the people is a matter of direct social concern.
(2) Social and economic conditions have an important effect on health and disease, and these relations must be the subject of scientific investigation.
(3) The measures taken to promote health and to contain disease must be social as well as medical.
(4) Medical statistics will be our standard of measurement.

Doctors are the natural advocates for the poor and the social questions fall for the most part in their jurisdiction. (Rudolf Virchow, *Medizinische Reform* (1948); Shepherd (1983) [8])

The public health approach is primarily concerned with the health of populations, not individuals. Although populations are clearly made up of individuals, the individual approach and the population approach are, in many ways, quite distinct. Measures of morbidity, explanations of possible causation, and the necessary interventions may be entirely different or require alternative strategies at these two levels.

Table 2.2 Changing definitions of community mental health services

G. F. Rehin and F. M. Martin (1963)

Any scheme directed to providing extra-mural care and treatment ... to facilitate the
early detection of mental health illness or relapse and its treatment on an informal
basis, and to provide some social work service in the community for support or
follow-up (quoted in Bennett and Freeman, 1991).

M. Sabshin (1966)

The utilisation of the techniques, methods, and theories of social psychiatry, as well as
those of the other behavioural sciences, to investigate and meet the mental health
needs of a functionally or geographically defined population over a significant period
of time, and the feeding back of information to modify the central body of social
mental health and other behavioural science and knowledge.

R. Freudenberg (1967)

Community psychiatry assumes that people with mental health disorders can be most
effectively helped when links with family, friends, workmates and society generally are
maintained, and aims to provide preventive, treatment, and rehabilitative services for a
district which means that therapeutic measures go beyond the individual patient.

G. Serban (1977)

Community psychiatry has three aspects: first, a social movement; second, a service
delivery strategy, emphasising the accessibility of services and acceptance of
responsibility of mental health needs of a total population; and third, provision of
best possible clinical care, with emphasis on the major mental health disorders and
on treatment outside total institutions.

D. Bennett (1978)

Community psychiatry is concerned with the mental health needs not only of the
individual patient, but of the district population, not only of those who are defined as
sick, but those who may be contributing to that sickness and whose health or wellbeing may, in turn, be put at risk.

M. Tansella (1986)

A system of care devoted to a defined population and based on a comprehensive and
integrated mental health service, which includes out-patient facilities, day and
residential training centres, residential accommodation in hostels, sheltered
workshops and in-patient units in general hospitals, and which ensures, with multi-
disciplinary team-work, early diagnosis, prompt treatment, continuity of care, social
support and a close liaison with other medical and social community services and, in
particular, with general practitioners.

G. Strathdee and G. Thornicroft (1997)

The network of services which offer continuing treatment, accommodation,
occupation and social support and which together help people with mental health
problems to regain their normal social roles.

G. Thornicroft and M. Tansella (1999)

A community-based mental health service is one which provides a full range of
effective mental health care to a defined population, and which is dedicated to
treating and helping people with mental disorders, in proportion to their suffering or
distress, in collaboration with other local agencies.

Table 2.3 Comparison of the public health and the individual health approaches

Public Health Approach	Individual Health Approach
(1) Whole population view	(1) Partial population view
(2) Patients seen in socio-economic context	(2) Tends to exclude contextual factors
(3) Interested in primary prevention	(3) Focus on treatment rather than prevention
(4) Individual as well as population-based interventions	(4) Individual level interventions only
(5) Service components seen in context of whole system	(5) Service components seen in isolation
(6) Favours open access to services on the basis of need	(6) Access to services on the basis of eligibility, e.g. by age, diagnosis or insurance cover
(7) Teamwork preferred	(7) Individual therapist preferred
(8) Long-term / life-course perspective	(8) Short-term and episodic perspective
(9) Cost-effectiveness seen in population terms	(9) Cost-effectiveness seen in individual terms

Psychiatrists, unlike sociologists, seem generally unaware of the existence and importance of mental health attributes of whole populations, their concern being only with sick individuals. (G. Rose, 1993 [9])

We wish to emphasise the need for mental-health practitioners to be able to understand, in addition to the individual-health approach, the public-health approach, and we compare the two in Table 2.3.

The needs of the mentally ill cannot safely be entrusted to the 'invisible hand' of market forces … mental health services should be based upon egalitarian principles, not simply as a moral imperative, but because a socially just system of provision is by far the most effective for a nation's health. (B. Cooper, 1995 [10])

The public health impact of mental disorders

The public health impact of mental disorders can be judged according to these criteria: (i) frequency; (ii) severity and consequences; (iii) availability of interventions and (iv) acceptability of interventions.

First, in terms of *frequency*, mental illnesses are common. Face-to-face household surveys of more than 60 000 adults in 2001–2003 in 40 countries worldwide, for example, showed that the prevalence of all mental disorders in the previous year varied, with most countries having rates between 9.1% and 16.1% [11;12]. More specifically, in the United States a national survey found that the prevalence rates of mental illness did not change between 1990 and 2003 [13]. By comparison, it is estimated that the total number of people with schizophrenia in less economically developed countries has increased from 16.7 million in 1985 to 24.4 million in 2000 [14], with continuing high proportions of people who are not treated, even in high-resource countries [12;15;16].

Second, as far as *severity* is concerned, mental illnesses can substantially interfere with life expectancy and with normal personal and social life [17–19]. In terms of mortality, such conditions contribute 8.1% of all *avoidable life years lost*, compared, for example, with 9% from respiratory diseases, 5.8% from all forms of cancer, and 4.4% from heart diseases [14;20]. In relation to *combined mortality and disability*, the World Bank has calculated this in terms of the Global Burden of Disease for different disorders, measured in disability-adjusted life years (DALY). These are defined as the sum of years of life lost because of premature mortality, plus the years of life lived with disability, adjusted for the severity of disability. An estimated 12% of worldwide DALYs are caused by psychiatric and behavioural disorders, exceeding even the global burden of cardiovascular conditions (9.7%) and malignant neoplasms (5.1%) [18;21]. By comparison, the average global expenditure on mental disorders is only 2% of national health budgets [18].

Depression, the most common mental disorder, is the leading cause of such global burden among all the mental illnesses. The proportion of all DALYs which are attributable to depression is expected to increase from 3.7% to 5.7% between 1990 and 2020, moving from 4th to 2nd in the overall ranking [22–25].

Mental disorders may also have important *consequences*, both for individuals with mental illness and for their families. For the individuals concerned, the consequences include the suffering caused by symptoms, lower quality of life, the loss of independence and work capacity, and poorer social integration [26–28]. For family members there is an increased burden from caring, and lowered economic productivity [17].

Third, as far as the *availability* of interventions is concerned, the public health approach implies that help should be made available and accessible, in proportion to need [29]. Interestingly, research suggests that usually this is not the case. In the large survey of mental illness conducted in the USA referred to above [13], the proportion of mentally ill people who received treatment rose from 20.3% to 32.9% between 1990 and 2003 [13]. Further, by 2003 only about half the people who received treatment had conditions that met diagnostic criteria, and so ran the risks of harm from unnecessary treatments with no prospect of benefit. This means that the health system in the USA has the capacity to treat up to two thirds of the people with clear-cut mental illnesses, but in fact only treats about one third. In other words, even in a very high-income country, most people with mental illness received no professional care. There is a paradox here. While mental disorders are very common, most people affected receive no treatment. Yet many people receiving treatment for mental illness are not actually mentally ill!

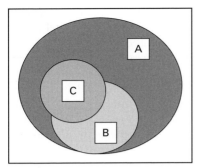

Figure 2.1 Relationship between true prevalence and treated prevalence. Key: A = total adult population, B = true prevalence, C = treated prevalence.

This raises the important issues of coverage and focusing. *Coverage* means the proportion of people that could benefit from treatment who actually receive it [30;31]. *Focusing* refers to how far those people actually receiving treatment in fact need it. In other words do they have any form of mental illness [32]? Even in the best resourced countries we find both low coverage and poor focusing. Within the European Region of the World Health Organisation an action plan calls on governments to provide effective care to people with mental illness [33–35]. Yet a comparative international study of depression found that 0% of depressed patients in St. Petersburg were treated with anti-depressants in primary care, and only 3% were referred on to specialist care. The inability of patients to afford out-of-pocket costs was the reason why 75% of the depressed Russian patients went untreated [36]. From the public health approach, therefore, the key issue is the appropriate use of resources, whatever the level of resources actually available, namely to increase both coverage and focus.

Figure 2.1 shows the relationship between true and treated prevalence. True prevalence means the total number of cases of a particular condition in a defined area. Treated prevalence, by contrast, refers to the fraction of this number of cases that are receiving care. In the National Comorbidity Survey Replication (NCS-R) study of 4319 participants representative of the general population in the USA (A, 100%), the true prevalence of all emotional disorders was 30.5% (B) of those surveyed, while 20.1% of all participants received treatment for any mental disorder (C) [13]. Among group C, half of these individuals did not have an emotional disorder at the time of treatment. Table 2.4 summarises this information numerically.

In a similar study in European countries (Belgium, France, Germany, Italy, Netherlands and Spain) using the same methods as the NCS-R, among 7731 participants, the true prevalence of all emotional disorders was 11.7%, and the

Table 2.4 National Comorbidity Survey Replication (NCS-R) data for true and treated annual prevalence rates of emotional disorders among adults in the general population

	Treated	Not treated	Total
Emotional disorder	10.07%	20.43%	30.50%
No emotional disorder	10.03%	59.47%	69.50%
Total	20.10%	79.90%	100%

Table 2.5 European rates of true and treated annual prevalence of emotional disorders among adults in the general population

	Treated	Not treated	Total
Emotional disorder	2.6%	9.1%	11.7% (true prevalence)
No emotional disorder	3.5%	84.8%	88.3%
Total	6.1% (treated prevalence)	93.9%	100%

treated rate was 6.1% of all respondents [37] (Table 2.5). Interestingly, among those who were treated, the majority had no disorder. Therefore in spite of the large differences in total prevalence rates between the USA and Europe, what mental health services share in common is an inability to focus their limited resources upon people who are actually mentally ill.

Fourth, in relation to *acceptability* of mental health services, three key issues are important: public knowledge about mental illness (usually very limited and characterised by ignorance or misinformation), public attitudes towards people with mental illnesses (largely fearful, indicating prejudice) and public behaviour towards both people with mental illness and mental health services (usually discriminatory) [38;39]. The extent of such stigmatising and discriminatory reactions show some cross-cultural differences, but their presence appears to be universal.

At the same time, there is accumulating evidence of successful interventions to reduce stigma [40;41]. At the national level, public awareness campaigns have so far shown some short-term improvements in, for example, knowledge and attitudes to depression [42;43]. At the local level, several intervention studies have shown the benefits of targeted educational interventions, for example for police officers or for school students, to reduce stigma [28;44–46]. Interestingly, the strongest evidence for what reduces stigma is that it is direct personal contact with people with mental illness at the individual level which makes a positive difference [38].

Prevention as a component of the public health approach

The public health approach offers a further distinct advantage in that it considers the *prevention* of disorders, not only their treatment. Although there is relatively little evidence that primary prevention of mental disorders has been effective on a widespread basis [47–49], the associations between social context and mental illnesses are well established. The quality of a person's social environment, for example, 'is closely linked to the risk for suffering a mental illness, to the triggering of an illness episode, and to the likelihood that such an illness will become chronic'. [14]

Poverty does appear to be a crucial factor in many of these complex relationships (see Figures 2.2 and 2.3). The association between low income and poor health, which is well established, may be either direct or indirect [50;51]. In fact, the cumulative impact of poverty may produce sustained effects upon physical, cognitive, psychological and social functioning [52–54].

Traditionally prevention has been described at three levels: primary, secondary and tertiary [55]. *Primary prevention* refers to measures which stop the onset of the condition. *Secondary prevention* refers to the early detection of people with a

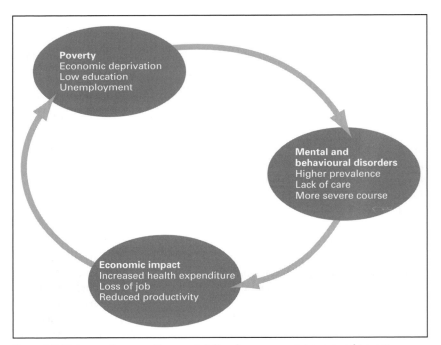

Figure 2.2 Vicious cycle connecting mental disorders, economic impact and poverty.
Source: World Health Organisation [18]. Reproduced with permission.

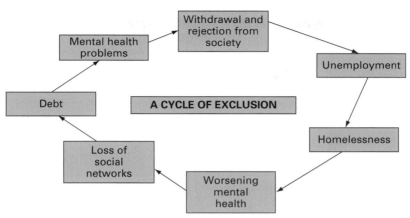

Figure 2.3 Complex relationships between mental illness and social exclusion.
Source: Social Exclusion Unit [26]. Reproduced with permission.

particular condition, usually by screening, where earlier treatment can significantly improve the course and outcome of the disorder. *Tertiary prevention* includes measures to reduce the disabling consequences of an already established condition. This framework is more useful in areas of health care in which causes are well identified, the time between the action of the causal factor and the onset of the condition is relatively short, there is a single primary cause, and where screening procedures are simple, effective and acceptable. Only the last of these criteria commonly applies to most mental disorders.

Another view is to see the three stages of prevention, treatment and rehabilitation as a continuum, and to define prevention in three ways: *universal, selected* and *indicated* [47–49]. *Universal* interventions are directed at the entire population and are less important at this stage of our limited knowledge about how to prevent mental illnesses. *Selected* interventions are targeted to individuals at risk, and since risk factors are more often identified than causes, in future we can expect increasing attention will be paid to such selected measures. *Indicated* interventions are directed to individuals at high risk, or to those with early features of illness.

In effect, the universal prevention approach is a *population-based strategy* [56] which aims to achieve prevention, not by targeting small numbers of high-risk individuals, but a far larger proportion of the population. The power of this strategy is that 'a large number of people exposed to a small risk commonly generates many more cases than a small number exposed to a high risk' [9]. In relation to mental disorders, this analysis would lead us to decrease population exposure to psycho-social or biological risk factors, not for only high-risk individuals, but for all members of the community. By contrast, prevention strategies which focus upon *high-risk individuals* attempt to reduce the impact of one or more risk factors for mental disorder.

The aims of the mental health service

It is now possible for us to set out the aims of the mental health service. In other words: what is its purpose? In terms of the matrix model, these aims can be described at the country, local and individual levels, as shown in Tables 2.6–2.8.

Conflicts may occur between different legitimate purposes of the mental health service. For example, there may be a direct conflict between an *individual's* need

Table 2.6 Mental health service aims at the national/regional level

- Receive information from the local level
- Combine and interpret data on particular problems, and to examine key associations (for example, between alcohol abuse and violence)
- Define a hierarchy of priorities
- Create a national strategic mental health plan
- Establish an implementation programme to put the national strategy into practice
- Monitor the working of local mental health services using an inspectorate system, rating services according to agreed standards and criteria
- Create, evaluate and disseminate treatment guidelines and protocols

Table 2.7 Mental health service aims at the local level

- Provide coverage by mental health services to those needing treatment
- Focus services only upon people able to benefit from treatment and care
- Improve the quality of treatment and care services, for example by assessing how far interventions are delivered in line with guidelines and protocols
- Collaborate with other local agencies to provide a network/system of care, for example, including links with primary care, and housing agencies
- Conduct selected and indicated prevention programmes
- Early detection of local changes in the nature or extent of mental disorders [57]

Table 2.8 Mental health service aims at the individual level

- Assess mental health needs
- Meet needs and remove symptoms if possible
- Ensure participation of people with mental illness (and their family members) in assessment, treatment and care
- Promote independence
- Provide information useful for individuals with mental illness and their family members
- Assist recovery and social participation
- Prevent relapse

for confidentiality of information, and the *local* need for other agencies to be aware of the identity of people with mental illness who have a history of violence. A second possible conflict is between the treatment choice (or treatment refusal) of an *individual* patient, and the demands of family members (or neighbours in the *local* area), if the person's behaviour becomes unacceptably disturbed. In this case the mental-health service may seek to fulfil two purposes simultaneously: to provide treatment and care to the person with mental illness, and to offer respite and protection for family members and others nearby.

Key points in this chapter

- 'Community care' means services close to home.
- A modern mental health service is a balance between community-based and hospital-based care.
- The public health approach is primarily concerned with the health of populations, not individuals.
- Mental illnesses contribute about 12% of the global burden of disease.
- Depression, the most common mental disorder, is the leading cause of global burden among all the mental illnesses.
- While mental disorders are very common, most people affected receive no treatment.
- Even in the best-resourced countries *coverage* rates are low (meaning the proportion of people that could benefit from treatment who actually receive it).
- Similarly services are often poorly *focused* (meaning how far those people who actually receive treatment really need it).

REFERENCES

1. Soanes C and Stevenson A. *Concise Oxford English Dictionary.* 11th edn. Oxford: Oxford University Press; 2003.
2. Ministry of Health. *Report on the Royal Commission on Mental Illness and Mental Deficiency.* London: HMSO; 1957.
3. Beer D, Jones E and Lipsedge M. History of psychiatric disorders and treatments. *Curr. Opin. Psychiatry* 2000; **13**: 709–715.
4. Bartlett P and Wright D. *The History of Care in the Community 1750–2000.* London: Athlone Press; 1999.
5. Bulmer M. *The Social Basis of Community Care.* London: Allen & Unwin; 1987.
6. Thornicroft G and Tansella M. Components of a modern mental health service: a pragmatic balance of community and hospital care: overview of systematic evidence. *Br. J. Psychiatry* 2004; **185**: 283–290.

7. Eisenberg L. Rudolf Ludwig Karl Virchow, where are you now that we need you? *Am. J. Med.* 1984; **77**(3): 524–532.

8. Shepherd M. The origins and directions of social psychiatry. *Integr. Psychiatry* 1983; September/October: 86–88.

9. Rose G. Mental disorder and the strategies of prevention. *Psychol. Med.* 1993; **23**: 553–555.

10. Cooper B. Do we still need social psychiatry? *Psychiatrica Fennica* 1995; **26**: 9–20.

11. Demyttenaere K, Bruffaerts R, Posada-Villa J, *et al.* Prevalence, severity, and unmet need for treatment of mental disorders in the World Health Organization World Mental Health Surveys. *JAMA* 2004; **291**(21): 2581–2590.

12. Wang PS, Guilar-Gaxiola S, Alonso J, *et al.* Use of mental health services for anxiety, mood, and substance disorders in 17 countries in the WHO world mental health surveys. *Lancet* 2007; **370**(9590): 841–850.

13. Kessler RC, Demler O, Frank RG, *et al.* Prevalence and treatment of mental disorders, 1990 to 2003. *N. Engl. J. Med.* 2005; **352**(24): 2515–2523.

14. Desjarlais R, Eisenberg L, Good B and Kleinman A. *World Mental Health. Problems and Priorities in Low Income Countries.* Oxford: Oxford University Press; 1995.

15. Thornicroft G. Most people with mental illness are not treated. *Lancet* 2007; **370** (9590): 807–808.

16. Saxena S, Thornicroft G, Knapp M and Whiteford H. Resources for mental health: scarcity, inequity, and inefficiency. *Lancet* 2007; **370**(9590): 878–889.

17. Thornicroft G, Tansella M, Becker T, *et al.* The personal impact of schizophrenia in Europe. *Schizophr. Res.* 2004; **69**(2–3): 125–132.

18. World Health Organisation. World Health Report 2001. *Mental Health: New Understanding, New Hope.* Geneva: World Health Organization; 2001.

19. Prince M, Patel V, Saxena S, *et al.* No health without mental health. *Lancet* 2007; **370** (9590): 859–877.

20. Harris EC and Barraclough B. Excess mortality of mental disorder. *Br. J. Psychiatry* 1998; **173**: 11–53.

21. Kohn R, Saxena S, Levav I and Saraceno B. Treatment gap in mental health care. *Bull. World Health Organ.* 2004; **82**: 858–866.

22. Murray C and Lopez A. *The Global Burden of Disease, Vol. 1. A Comprehensive Assessment of Mortality and Disability from Diseases, Injuries and Risk Factors in 1990, and Projected to 2020.* Cambridge, MA: Harvard University Press; 1996.

23. Moussavi S, Chatterji S, Verdes E, *et al.* Depression, chronic diseases, and decrements in health: results from the World Health Surveys. *Lancet* 2007; **370**(9590): 851–858.

24. Chisholm D, Flisher A, Lund C, *et al.* Scale up services for mental disorders: a call for action. *Lancet* 2007; **370**(9594): 1241–1252.

25. Chisholm D, Sanderson K, Yuso-Mateos JL and Saxena S. Reducing the global burden of depression: population-level analysis of intervention cost-effectiveness in 14 world regions. *Br. J. Psychiatry* 2004; **184**: 393–403.

26. Social Exclusion Unit. *Mental Health and Social Exclusion.* London: Office of the Deputy Prime Minister; 2004.

27. Sayce L and Curran C. Tackling social exclusion across Europe. In Knapp M, McDaid D, Mossialos E and Thornicroft G (Eds.). *Mental Health Policy and*

Practice Across Europe. The Future Direction of Mental Health Care. Milton Keynes: Open University Press; 2006.

28. Sartorius N and Schulze H. *Reducing the Stigma of Mental Illness. A Report From a Global Programme of the World Psychiatric Association.* Cambridge: Cambridge University Press; 2005.

29. Thornicroft G, Becker T, Knapp M, *et al. International Outcome Measures in Mental Health. Quality of Life, Needs, Service Satisfaction, Costs and Impact on Carers.* London: Gaskell, Royal College of Psychiatrists; 2005.

30. Habicht JP, Mason JP and Tabatabai H. Basic concepts for the design of evaluations during programme implementation. In Sahn D R, Lockwood R and Scrimshaw N S (Eds.). *Methods for the Evaluation of the Impact of Food and Nutrition Programmes. Food and Nutrition Bulletin.* Suppl. 8. New York: The United Nations University; 1984. 1–25.

31. Alonso J, Codony M, Kovess V, *et al.* Population level of unmet need for mental healthcare in Europe. *Br. J. Psychiatry* 2007; **190**: 299–306.

32. Tansella M. Recent advances in depression. Where are we going? *Epidemiologia e Psichiatria Sociale* 2006; **15**: 1–3.

33. World Health Organisation. *Mental Health Action Plan for Europe.* Copenhagen: World Health Organisation; 2005.

34. World Health Organisation. *Mental Health Declaration for Europe.* Copenhagen: World Health Organisation; 2005.

35. Thornicroft G and Rose D. Mental health in Europe. *BMJ* 2005; **330**(7492): 613–614.

36. Simon GE, Fleck M, Lucas R and Bushnell DM. Prevalence and predictors of depression treatment in an international primary care study. *Am. J. Psychiatry* 2004; **161**(9): 1626–1634.

37. Alonso J and Lepine JP, the ESEMeD/MHEDEA 2000 Scientific Committee. Overview of the key ESEMeD data. *J. Clin. Psychiatry* 2007; **68**(Suppl. 2): 3–9.

38. Thornicroft G. *Shunned: Discrimination against People with Mental Illness.* Oxford: Oxford University Press; 2006.

39. Thornicroft G. Stigma and discrimination limit access to mental health care. *Epidemiol. Psichiatr. Soc.* 2008;(17): in press.

40. Pinfold V, Thornicroft G, Huxley P and Farmer P. Active ingredients in anti-stigma programmes in mental health. *Int. Rev. Psychiatry* 2005; **17**(2): 123–131.

41. Thornicroft G, Rose D, Kassam A and Sartorius N. Stigma: ignorance, prejudice or discrimination? *Br. J. Psychiatry* 2007; **190**: 192–193.

42. Jorm AF, Christensen H and Griffiths KM. The impact of Beyondblue: the national depression initiative on the Australian public's recognition of depression and beliefs about treatments. *Aust. N. Z. J. Psychiatry* 2005; **39**(4): 248–254.

43. Hickie I. Can we reduce the burden of depression? The Australian experience with Beyondblue: the national depression initiative. *Australas Psychiatry* 2004; **12** Suppl: S38–S46.

44. Schulze B, Richter-Werling M, Matschinger H and Angermeyer MC. Crazy? So what! Effects of a school project on students' attitudes towards people with schizophrenia. *Acta Psychiatr. Scand.* 2003; **107**(2): 142–150.

45. Pinfold V, Huxley P, Thornicroft G, *et al.* Reducing psychiatric stigma and discrimination – evaluating an educational intervention with the police force in England. *Soc. Psychiatry Psychiatr. Epidemiol.* 2003; **38**(6): 337–344.

46. Pinfold V, Toulmin H, Thornicroft G, *et al.* Reducing psychiatric stigma and discrimination: evaluation of educational interventions in UK secondary schools. *Br. J. Psychiatry* 2003; **182**: 342–346.

47. Hosman C, Jane-Llopis E and Saxena S. *Prevention of Mental Disorders: Effective Interventions and Policy Options.* Oxford: Oxford University Press; 2005.

48. Jane-Llopis E, Hosman C, Jenkins R and Anderson P. Predictors of efficacy in depression prevention programmes. Meta-analysis. *Br. J. Psychiatry* 2003; **183**: 384–397.

49. Hosman C, Jane-Llopis E and Saxena S. *Prevention of Mental Disorders.* Geneva: World Health Organization; 2004.

50. Marmot M. The influence of income on health: views of an epidemiologist. *Health Aff. (Millwood)* 2002; **21**(2): 31–46.

51. Warr P. *Work, Unemployment and Mental Health.* Oxford: Oxford University Press; 1987.

52. Lynch JW, Kaplan GA and Salonen JT. Why do poor people behave poorly? Variation in adult health behaviours and psychosocial characteristics by stages of the socioeconomic lifecourse. *Soc. Sci. Med.* 1997; **44**(6): 809–819.

53. Patel V, Araya R, Chatterjee S, *et al.* Treatment and prevention of mental disorders in low-income and middle-income countries. *Lancet* 2007; **370**(9591): 991–1005.

54. Patel V, Farooq S and Thara R. What is the best approach to treating schizophrenia in developing countries? *PLoS Med.* 2007; **4**(6): e159.

55. Newton J. *Preventing Mental Illness in Practice.* London: Routledge; 1992.

56. Rose G. *The Strategy of Preventive Medicine.* Oxford: Oxford University Press; 1992.

57. Cooper B. Single spies and battalions: the clinical epidemiology of mental disorders. *Psychol. Med.* 1993; **23**: 891–907.

3

The historical context

We present here only a highly selective account of the historical context, as several excellent analyses have already been published [1–8]. The history of mental health care over about the last century in the more economically developed nations can be described in relation to *three historical periods*. Period 1 describes the rise of the asylum, between about 1880 and 1950; Period 2 is the decline of the asylum, from around 1950 to 1980; and Period 3 refers to the development of decentralised, community-based mental health care, since approximately 1980. These three periods are summarised in Tables 3.1–3.3. The dates applicable to each period vary considerably between different countries and regions. Viewing these changes in a longer-term perspective, the development of community-based services is in fact a very recent historical phenomenon.

Key transitions in this historical process have often been triggered by scandals. A series of inquiries, for example, into malpractice at several British hospitals for the mentally ill provided the occasion for critical evaluation of such institutions. The recurring themes from inquires into the causes of ill-treatment have been identified: isolation of the institutions, lack of staff support, poor reporting procedures, a failure of leadership, ineffective administration, inadequate financial resources, the divided loyalties of trade unions, poor staff training and occasional negligent individuals [9].

Period 1. The rise of the asylum (1880–1950)

Period 1, the rise of the asylum, occurred between approximately 1880 and 1950 in many of the more economically developed countries. It was characterised by the construction and enlargement of asylums, remote from the original homes of patients, offering mainly custodial containment and the provision of the basic necessities for survival, to people with a wide range of clinical and social abnormalities. The asylums therefore acted as repositories for those considered untreatable or socially deviant.

Table 3.1 The key characteristics of three periods in the historical development of mental health systems of care

Period 1 (1880–1950)	Period 2 (1950–1980)	Period 3 (Since 1980)
Asylums built	Asylums neglected	Asylums replaced by smaller facilities
Increasing number of beds	Decreasing number of beds	Decrease in the number of beds slows down
Reduced role for the family	Increasing, but not fully recognised, role of the family	Importance of families increasingly recognised, in terms of care given, therapeutic potential, the burden carried, and as a political lobbying group
Public investment in institutions	Public disinvestment in mental health services	Increasing private investment in treatment and care, and focus in public sector on cost-effectiveness and cost containment.
Staff: doctors and nurses only	Clinical psychologist, occupational therapists and social worker disciplines evolve Effective treatments emerge, beginning of treatment evaluation and of standardised diagnostic systems, growing influence of individual and group psychotherapy	More community-based staff, and emphasis on multi-disciplinary team working Emergence of 'evidence-based' psychiatry in relation to pharmacological, social and psychological treatments
Primacy of containment over treatment	Focus on pharmacological control and social rehabilitation, fewer disabled patients discharged from asylums	Emergence of concern about balance between control of patients and their independence

In economic terms, this required considerable investment, and large institutions were built in the last two decades of the nineteenth century in many countries. Indeed the choice of remote sites fitted both the need to physically remove this perceived threat to the public safety, and was also consistent with current views of mental hygiene, which held that recovery was facilitated by restful country settings. One consequence of this choice of geographical location was the subsequent professional segregation of psychiatrists and nurses from the main body of clinical practice, and from the centres of professional status in the metropolitan, university teaching hospitals.

Table 3.2 Geographical levels of the matrix model and the differential historical development of mental health systems

Geographical Level	Period 1 (1880–1950)	Period 2 (1950–1980)	Period 3 (Since 1980)
Country / Regional	Emphasis on concentration of undifferentiated patients (the indigent, mentally or physically handicapped, demented, and psychotic) in single remote mental hospitals, where patients were categorised by behaviour and sex	Larger asylums retain differentiated responsibility for the long-stay patients: including the more behaviourally disturbed, or treatment non-responsive, and mentally handicapped. Differentiation of specialist wards / hospitals for forensic patients	Decreasing number of adult long-stay beds in health service facilities. Remaining regional level facilities focus on forensic services
Local		Beginning of psychiatric wards in general hospitals for acute patients, differentiated from day hospital, day centre, sheltered workshops, and other local rehabilitation facilities	Increasing number of community mental health teams and centres. Proliferation of local non-hospital residential facilities, including hostels, group homes, nursing homes, sheltered apartments, and supported housing schemes. Decreasing emphasis upon separate rehabilitation facilities
Individual			Design of individualised inter-agency treatment programmes involving multi-disciplinary teams, voluntary organisations, GPs, social services, church and charities etc. Less separation between treatment and rehabilitation, stress on secondary prevention of relapse, and also on improving quality of life More evidence-based psychotherapies

Table 3.3 Temporal phases of the matrix model and the differential historical development of mental health systems of care

Phases	Period 1 (1880–1950)	Period 2 (1950–1980)	Period 3 (Since 1980)
Inputs	Attention primarily upon buildings. Poor staff selection and training, mental health and social welfare legislation to regulate the use of institutions	Building of occupational and rehabilitation centres, modernisation of legal and policy framework, development of liaison between psychiatry and other medical disciplines, establishment of newer allied disciplines, and sub-specialities within psychiatry. New anti-psychotic and anti-depressant medications	Community mental health centres built, individual, family and population-level needs assessments, home treatment teams, new anti-depressant and anti-psychotic medications, integrated pharmacological and psycho-social treatments, cognitive-behavioural treatment, self-help and patient advocacy, modernisation of mental health legislation in some countries. Enhanced attention from mass media. Emphasis on the control of public expenditure
Processes		Influence of psychodynamic theory on mental health services at zenith. Decreasing length of in-patient stay and appearance of 'revolving door' pattern of service use. Reduced bed numbers in asylums, but hospital costs not reduced. Diversion of acute patients to acute hospitals. Attention to group processes in 'therapeutic milieu', therapeutic communities, and group psychotherapy. Monitoring patterns of service contact using case registers	Focus on continuity of care over time, by the same team, and/or co-ordination between different agencies, using, for example, case management. Targeting services toward more disabled patients. Greater attention to risk assessment. Development of audit of clinical practice. Growth of evaluative research as a tool to improve clinical practice. Introduction of market principles (separation of purchaser and provider roles, designed to improve quality through competition)
Outcomes			At the country and local levels limited use of indicators (mortality, suicide and homelessness rates). At the individual level standardised outcomes measures in research studies, and in some clinical services, rated by staff, service-users and their families

---

asylum *noun*

(1) sanctuary; protection, esp. for those pursued by the law (*seek asylum*)

(2) *historical.* any of various kinds of institution offering shelter and support to distressed or destitute individuals, esp. the mentally ill

Source: Concise Oxford Dictionary (1993)

Three themes were apparent throughout these developments namely: clinical, humanitarian and economic considerations. In 1842 the English Poor Law Commissioners, for example, reported that '[i]t must, however, be remembered that with lunatics, the first object ought to be their cure by means of proper medical treatment.' (Poor Law Commission, 1842).

The economic argument was also given early prominence. In 1838 Edward Gulson, Assistant Poor Law Commissioner, gave evidence to the House of Commons Select Committee on the Poor Law Amendment Act. He recommended a transfer of power over lunatics from the county asylums to the Poor Law Commissioners, 'where they would be kept at one half or a third or a fourth of the expense at which they are now kept'. These three guiding imperatives, the clinical, the moral and the financial, therefore combined in a subtle and continuing interplay, the effects of which were manifest in the late nineteenth century as the establishment and overgrowth of the asylums. Interestingly current critics of community care still often refer to such polices as primarily intended to cut costs.

Gli infermieri non devono tenere relazioni con le famiglie dei malati, darne notizia, portare fuori senz'ordine lettere, oggetti, ambasciate, saluti: ne' possono recare agli ammalati alcuna notizia dal di fuori, ne' oggetti, ne' stampe, ne' scritti. (Norma di regolamento in un ospedale psichiatrico)

Nurses must not have relationships with families of patients, pass on information, take out of the hospital without orders letters, objects, messages, greetings: nor are they allowed to bring to patients any news from outside, or objects, or printed material or notes. (From a list of regulations in a psychiatric hospital)

Quoted in *Morire di classe, a cura di Franco Basaglia e Franca Basaglia Ongaro. La condizione manicomiale fotografata by Carla Cerati and Gianni Berengo Gardin.* Einaudi, Torino 1969.

It is important to note that although we suggest that the three historical periods have occurred consecutively, the times at which they began and finished in different countries have varied greatly. In Italy, for example, psychiatric bed numbers were stable until 1963 [10], and then diminished precipitously after the legislation introduced in 1978, so it is reasonable to conclude that in Italy Period 1 began about a decade later than in England.

Notably, until the Italian mental heath law of 1978, the responsibility for both public and private asylums lay not with the Health Ministry, but with the

Ministry of Internal Affairs and its local prefectures. Similarly, until 1968 everyone who had been admitted to a psychiatric hospital had their names entered by a tribunal into a national judicial register, which was a lifelong assignment (which also persisted after hospital discharge), and this was considered a shameful family stigma which meant the permanent loss of many civil rights, including voting, and the ownership of property and land.

Although we suggest a three-stage sequence of historical events, in fact later developmental stages will often retain remnants of earlier times. For example, a few remaining large and remote vestigial institutions, in which poor material and treatment conditions survived, may have continued after the development of community care, especially in sub-specialist areas such as forensic psychiatry. In Japan, for example, the number of beds in 1960 was 95 067, and this increased to 172 950 in 1965. By 1993 there were 1672 psychiatric hospitals which contained 362 963 beds, a degree of in-patient provision far higher than in most economically developed nations. There has been a slight decrease in bed numbers since 1993 [11;12].

Period 2. The decline of the asylum (1950–1980)

The rationale for deinstitutionalisation and the justification for the transfer of long-stay patients from the larger psychiatric hospitals are based on sociological, pharmacological, administrative and legal changes [5;8]. From the mid 1950s an increasingly forceful sociological opinion emerged. This view criticised the ill effects of prolonged stay within large psychiatric institutions. Goffman formulated the concept of the 'total institution', central to which was 'the handling of many human needs by the bureaucratic organisation of whole blocks of people' [13]. Wing and Brown reinforced this view with their description of the 'institutionalism' of chronic patients. From their study of long-stay patients in three British hospitals, they accepted the hypothesis that 'the social conditions under which a patient lives (particularly poverty of the social environment) are actually responsible for part of the symptomatology (particularly the negative symptoms)' [14].

Treatment patterns were also changing rapidly. Within three years of the formulation of chlorpromazine in 1952, its use as an anti-psychotic agent was widespread [1]. The decline of asylums is often reported in association with the 'anti-psychotic drugs revolution'. While we fully recognise the usefulness of these drugs, their importance should not obscure other revolutionary innovations in patient care. Industrial Therapy Organisations, for example, were set up; therapeutic communities were developed; day hospitals appeared; hostels and half-way houses were established.

As far as anti-psychotic drugs are concerned, it was evident from the outset that while their impact on psychiatric practice was considerable, the view that the coincident fall in the resident population of mental hospitals was directly due to their introduction was subject to considerable controversy. At the first International Collegium of Neuro-Psychopharmacology (ICNP), Sir Aubrey Lewis reported that 'British figures regarding mental hospital populations impose caution in giving the pharmacological action of these new drugs most of the credit for the undoubted fall that has occurred in the absolute number of people resident in certain mental hospitals' [15]. Shortly afterwards, Shepherd and colleagues published a statistical account of the changes in an English county mental hospital before and after the introduction of the psychotropic drugs in 1955, which proved that the impact of pharmacotherapy was very small, and suggested that the non-specific benefits of new drugs may already have been attained by other measures, such as more medical personnel, changing criteria for discharge, increased acceptance of the mentally ill by families and by the community, and the expansion of rehabilitative practices and social facilities [16].

> Certainly if we had to choose between abandoning the use of all the new psychotropic drugs and abandoning the Industrial Resettlement Units and other social facilities available to us, there would be no hesitation about the choice: the drugs would go. (Sir Aubrey Lewis, 1959 [15])

Financial considerations have also been especially important in fostering this transfer of care. In the United States, for example, the introduction of Medicaid in the 1960s promoted a rapid expansion of nursing homes with an associated transfer of financial responsibility, or 'cost shifting', from state to federal programmes [17].

For much of this time deinstitutionalisation had been left undefined. In 1975 the then Director of the National Institute of Mental Health in the USA, described three essential components of such an approach: the prevention of inappropriate mental hospital admissions through the provision of community facilities; the release to the community of all institutional patients who have received adequate preparation; and the establishment and maintenance of community support systems for non-institutionalised patients. A more succinct definition was the contraction of traditional institutional settings, with the concurrent expansion of community-based services [17].

In Italy, the maximum number of psychiatric beds occurred in 1963 (91 868 residents, 1.61 per 1000 population), and by 1981 the number had more than halved (38 358, 0.68 per 1000 population). During this same period the number of admissions grew steadily until 1975, three years before the reform of 1978, which made first admissions to traditional large mental hospitals illegal (in fact since 1982 all admissions to these institutions, both public and private, have been against the law). In this respect Italy is atypical compared with other

Western European countries, which have continued to rely to some extent upon these longer-stay hospitals as a last resort.

> The average standard of psychiatric practice in Britain is abysmally low. Psychiatrists themselves are sometimes reluctant to make this admission, though the evidence is overwhelming. In an average mental hospital a long-stay patient is likely to see a doctor for only ten minutes or so every three months … Scandals about the ill treatment of patients in mental hospitals, including those of relatively good reputation, occur with monotonous regularity. (Anthony Clare (1976) [18])

Period 3. Developing community care (since 1980)

We do not wish to suggest that the historical development of mental-health services is a consistent linear trend from the asylum to community-based system of care [19]. Rather there are oscillations which have been described as 'cycles of care' [20]. Indeed intriguing parallels appear when we compare the central themes of nineteenth- and twentieth-century mental health services, as summarised in Table 3.4.

Across the European continent as a whole, very similar changes have taken place, although to different timescales. There is now a clear divide between the countries of Western Europe, which have largely completed the process of deinstitutionalisation, and the position in most Central and Eastern European states, in which the transition from institutional care to a more balanced mix of services is only now starting [21–24] (see Figures 3.1 and 3.2 [25]). At its worst, the challenges of institutional practices (persisting from totalitarian times), very

Table 3.4 Parallels between late nineteenth- and late twentieth-century developments

Phase	Nineteenth century	Twentieth century
Optimism phase	Mental hygiene movement	Community mental health approach
Building phase	Institutions: large, mental hospitals, operating as self-sufficient and isolated communities	Decentralised community mental health centres and smaller residential and day-care facilities
Disillusionment phase	Overcrowding of accumulating patients	Scandals, inquiries and public reaction
Control phase	Attempt to differentiate between 'curable' and 'incurable' patients	Attempt to differentiate between 'safe' and 'risk' patients

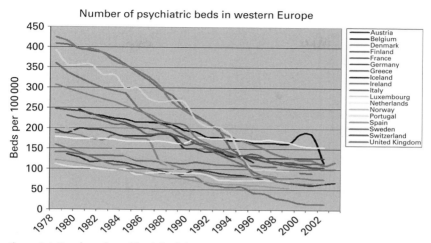

Figure 3.1 Number of psychiatric beds in Western Europe.

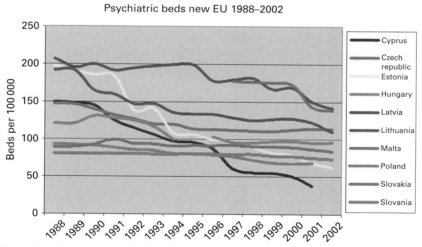

Figure 3.2 Number of psychiatric beds in new EU 1988–2002.

low funding levels, and remote locations have led to severe abuses of human rights at mental hospitals in several Eastern European countries [26–28]. At the global level two new systems that monitor and track mental health service across the world have recently been introduced by the World Health Organisation, called ATLAS and AIMS [29–32].

As for the future development of mental health services? '... the predictions of the future are usually statements of current desires; and the methods which are proposed to achieve goals in the future have the limitation of the past, when they were produced.' [33]

Key points in this chapter

- Recent history of mental-health care in the more economically developed nations is described in relation to three *historical periods*; (i) the rise of the asylum; (ii) the decline of the asylum; (iii) the development of decentralised, community-based mental health care.
- Justification for the transfer of long-stay patients from the larger psychiatric hospitals are based on sociological, pharmacological, administrative and legal changes.
- Deinstitutionalisation has been defined as the contraction of traditional institutional settings, with the concurrent expansion of community-based services.
- Cycles of care often pass through four stages: optimism; building; disillusionment and control.
- At the global level two new systems that monitor and track mental health services across the world have recently been introduced by the World Health Organisation, called ATLAS and AIMS.

REFERENCES

1. Jones K. *A History of Mental Health Services*. London: Routledge and Kegan Paul; 1972.
2. Scull A. *Decarceration*. New Jersey: Prentice-Hall; 1977.
3. Gilman SL. *Seeing the Insane*. Wiley: New York; 1982.
4. Grob G. *From Asylum to Community. Mental Health Policy in Modern America*. Princeton, NJ: Princeton University Press; 1991.
5. Shorter E. *A History of Psychiatry: From the Era of the Asylum to the Age of Prozac*. New York: John Wiley & Sons, Inc.; 1997.
6. Thornicroft G and Tansella M. *The Mental Health Matrix: A Manual to Improve Services*. Cambridge: Cambridge University Press; 1999.
7. Shorter E. *Historical Dictionary of Psychiatry*. Oxford: Oxford University Press; 2005.
8. Shorter E. The historical development of mental health services in Europe. In Knapp M, McDaid D, Mossialos E and Thornicroft G (Eds.). *Mental Health Policy and Practice Across Europe*. Buckingham: Open University Press; 2007. 15–33.
9. Martin S. *Hospitals in Trouble*. London: Blackwell; 1985.

10. Tansella M, De Salvia D and Williams P. The Italian psychiatric reform: some quantitative evidence. *Soc. Psychiatry* 1987; **22**(1): 37–48.

11. Oshima I, Mino Y and Inomata Y. Institutionalisation and schizophrenia in Japan: social environments and negative symptoms: nationwide survey of in-patients. *Br. J. Psychiatry* 2003; **183**: 50–56.

12. Oshima I, Mino Y and Inomata Y. How many long-stay schizophrenia patients can be discharged in Japan? *Psychiatry Clin Neurosci* 2007; **61**(1): 71–77.

13. Goffman I. *Asylums*. Harmondsworth: Pelican Books; 1968.

14. Wing JK and Brown G. *Institutionalism and Schizophrenia*. Cambridge: Cambridge University Press; 1970.

15. Lewis A. The impact of psychotropic drugs on the structure, function and future of psychiatric services in hospitals. In Bradley P, Deniker P and Raduco-Thomas C (Eds.). *Neuropsychopharmacology*. Amsterdam: Elsevier; 1959. 207.

16. Shepherd M, Goodman N and Watt D. The application of hospital statistics in the evaluation of pharmacotherapy in a psychiatric population. *Compr. Psychiatry* 1961; **2**: 11–19.

17. Bachrach L. *Deinstitutionalization: An Analytical Review and Sociological Perspective*. Rockville, MD: US Department of Health, Education and Welfare; 1976.

18. Clare A. *Psychiatry in Dissent*. London: Routledge; 1976.

19. Thornicroft G and Bebbington P. Deinstitutionalisation – from hospital closure to service development. *Br. J. Psychiatry* 1989; **155**: 739–753.

20. Morrissey JP and Goldman HH. Cycles of reform in the care of the chronically mentally ill. *Hosp. Community Psychiatry* 1984; **35**(8): 785–793.

21. Tomov T. Central and Eastern European Countries. In Thornicroft G and Tansella M (Eds.). *The Mental Health Matrix. A Manual to Improve Services*. Cambridge: Cambridge University Press; 2001. 216–227.

22. World Health Organisation. Mental Health in Europe. *Country Reports from the WHO European Network on Mental Health*. Copenhagen: World Health Organisation; 2001.

23. Thornicroft G and Tansella M. Components of a modern mental health service: a pragmatic balance of community and hospital care: overview of systematic evidence. *Br. J. Psychiatry* 2004; **185**: 283–290.

24. Thornicroft G and Rose D. Mental health in Europe. *BMJ* 2005; **330**(7492): 613–614.

25. Knapp MJ, McDaid D, Mossialos E and Thornicroft G. *Mental Health Policy and Practice Across Europe*. Buckingham: Open University Press; 2005.

26. Amnesty International. *Memorandum to the Romanian Government Concerning Inpatient Psychiatric Treatment*. London: Amnesty International; 2004.

27. Mental Disability Advocacy Center. *Cage Beds*. Budapest: Mental Disability Advocacy Centre; 2003.

28. Tomov T, van Voren R, Keukens R and Puras D. Mental health policy in former eastern bloc countries. In Knapp M, McDaid D, Mossialos E and Thornicroft G (Eds.). *Mental Health Policy and Practice across Europe*. Buckingham: Open University Press; 2007.

29. World Health Organisation. *Mental Health Atlas 2001*. Geneva: World Health Organisation; 2001.

30. World Health Organisation. *Mental Health Atlas 2005*. Geneva: World Health Organisation; 2005.

31. Saxena S, Sharan P, Garrido M and Saraceno B. World Health Organization's Mental Health Atlas 2005: implications for policy development. *World Psychiatry* 2006; **5**(3): 179–184.

32. World Health Organisation. *World Health Organisation Assessment Instrument for Mental Health Systems (WHO-AIMS)*. Geneva: World Health Organisation; 2005.

33. Sartorius N. Experience from the mental health programme of the World Health Organization. *Acta Psychiatr. Scand. Suppl.* 1988; **344**: 71–74.

4

The ethical base for mental health care

Intellect has a keen eye for method and technique but is blind to aim and value.
(Albert Einstein)

The following three chapters will discuss the contributions of *ethics*, *evidence*, and *experience* to the complex issues of mental health care improvement. This sequence is intentional because we believe that these three aspects should be seen hierarchically. We place ethics first as we consider that in health care there is no place for interventions which are technically effective, but which are unethical. In relation to biomedical ethics as a whole, four principles have been described as the foundations of medical ethics: respect for autonomy, non-maleficence, beneficence, and justice [1–3].

Principles are important because they can guide and shape decisions about the general organisation and specific daily activities of mental health care. Even if these ethical issues are not made explicit in planning and service delivery, they will exert a profound influence on clinical practice. In our view it is better to make the ethical framework explicit early in a planning cycle, because if such discussions are not held openly among all relevant groups, then fundamental disagreements on what mental health services should be trying to achieve will become manifest in other, and usually more destructive, ways. Indeed, it is our experience that when discussions on principles do not take place, then value conflicts will anyway occur sooner or later, and may then slow, limit or even completely undermine the viability of any plans. We shall now discuss the place of ethics at the national, local and individual levels.

Guiding principles at the national level

People with mental illnesses in many countries are treated in ways which prevent them from exercising some of their basic human rights. It is hardly an exaggeration to say that we can estimate the value attached to people with mental illness quite precisely from seeing how much or how little attention is paid to ensuring that they are treated in fully humane ways [4]. Several legally binding conventions and declarations apply to disabled people in general and to people with mental health-related disabilities in particular [5;6]. These international agreements apply to all nation states which have formally ratified them.

> All persons have the right to the best available mental heath care, which shall be part of the health and social care system. (Mental Illness Principle of the United Nations International Covenant on Economic, Social and Cultural Rights[7])

The primary source of international human rights within the United Nations (UN) is the Universal Declaration of Human Rights (UDHR), which refers to civil, political, economic, social and cultural rights. Civil and political rights, such as the right to liberty, to a fair trial and to vote, are set out in an internationally binding treaty, the International Covenant on Civil and Political Rights (ICCPR). Economic, social and cultural rights, such as the rights to an adequate standard of living, the highest attainable standard of physical and mental health, and to education, are described in a second binding treaty, the International Covenant on Economic, Social and Cultural Rights (ICESCR). The United Nations High Commissioner for Human Rights (UNHCHR) reports to the UN on the implementation of these principles. Countries which have ratified this declaration and this convention are then obliged under international law to guarantee to every person on their territory, without discrimination, all the rights agreed [7–11].

More specifically in relation to mental illness, the UN Principles for the Protection of Persons with Mental Illness and for the Improvement of Mental-Health Care were adopted in 1991, and elaborate the basic rights and freedoms of people with mental illness that must be secured if states are to be in full compliance with the ICESCR. 'The Right to Mental Health' is stated in Article 12 of the ICESCR, which recognises 'the right of everyone to the enjoyment of the highest attainable standard of physical and mental health', and identifies some of the measures states should take 'to achieve the full realisation of this right'.

These Mental Illness Principles apply to all people with mental illness, whether or not in in-patient psychiatric care, and to all people admitted to psychiatric facilities, whether or not they are diagnosed as having a mental illness. They provide criteria for the determination of mental illness, protection of confidentiality, standards of care, the rights of people in mental health facilities, and the provision of resources.

Mental Illness Principle 1 lays down the basic foundation upon which states' obligations towards people with mental illness are built: that 'all persons with a mental illness, or who are being treated as such persons, shall be treated with humanity and respect for the inherent dignity of the human person', and 'shall have the right to exercise all civil, political, economic, social and cultural rights as recognised in the Universal Declaration of Human Rights, the International

Covenant on Economic, Social and Cultural Rights, the International Covenant on Civil and Political Rights and in other relevant instruments'. It also provides that 'all persons have the right to the best available mental health care'. As the United Nations' health agency, the World Health Organisation (WHO) reflects the UN's understanding of what is meant by 'the best available mental health care' [12].

In addition to these global agreements, 43 member states of the Council of Europe are bound by particular human rights principles [13;14]. These include the 1950 European Convention on Human Rights and Fundamental Freedoms (ECHR), and the European Convention for the Prevention of Torture and Inhuman or Degrading Treatment or Punishment. Table 4.2 shows 12 principles which appear most often among such policy documents [15].

The Pan American Health Organisation / WHO Regional Office for the Americas has issued the Caracas Declaration which sets out the principles relevant in modernising mental health care in Latin America (see Table 4.1), which was later evaluated in relation to the Principles of Brazilia [16].

By now it is perhaps becoming clear to you that there is no international consensus on which principles should guide health care, let alone mental health care. Rather there are many systems which have been devised by different groups at different times [5;12;18–20]. To some extent many of these declarations are rather similar and Table 4.2 identifies 12 common themes.

Nevertheless, in our view it is both important to make a clear statement about which values guide any given service development, and to give careful thought to which specific principles are selected for that particular purpose and at that particular time. One example of the need for specifically tailored principles is those chosen for a new mental health law in South Africa, after the end of the apartheid, as shown in Table 4.3.

Another example of the use of such abstractions is the way that value and principles were incorporated into the national mental health plan for England after widespread consultation with many stakeholder groups (see Table 4.4).

Guiding principles at the local level

We have selected nine principles, described in detail in a previous book [26], which refer to developing local mental health services, as shown in Table 4.5. While there may be some degree of overlap between them, they are largely distinct and can be applied to a very wide range of circumstances, and from their initials can be called the 'Three Aces'! [27]

Of these nine principles, four are particularly relevant for local services: accessibility, comprehensiveness, continuity and co-ordination.

Table 4.1 Summary of Declaration of Caracas 1990 [17]

The legislators, associations, health authorities, mental health professionals and jurists assembled at the Regional Conference on the Restructuring of Psychiatric Care in Latin America within the Local Health Systems Model declare:

(1) That the restructuring of psychiatric care on the basis of Primary Health Care and within the framework of the Local Health Systems Model will promote alternative service models that are community-based and integrated into social and health care networks.

(2) That the restructuring of psychiatric care in the Region implies a critical review of the dominant and centralizing role played by the mental hospital in mental health service delivery.

(3) That the resources, care and treatment that are made available must:
    (a) safeguard personal dignity and human and civil rights;
    (b) be based on criteria that are rational and technically appropriate; and
    (c) strive to maintain patients in their communities.

(4) That national legislation must be redrafted if necessary so that:
    (a) the human and civil rights of mental patients are safeguarded; and
    (b) that the organization of community mental health services guarantees the protection of these rights.

(5) That training in mental health and psychiatry should use a service model that is based on the community health center and encourages psychiatric admission in general hospitals, in accordance with the principles that underlie the restructuring movement.

(6) That the organizations, associations, and other participants in this Conference hereby undertake to advocate and develop programs at the country level that will promote the desired restructuring, and at the same time commit themselves to monitoring and defending the human rights of mental patients in accordance with the national legislation and international agreements.

   To this end, they call upon the Ministries of Health and Justice, the Parliaments, Social Security and other care-providing institutions, professional organizations, consumer associations, universities and other training facilities and the media to support the restructuring of psychiatric care, thus assuring this successful development for the benefit of the population in the Region.

Accessibility

The central point about accessibility is that people should be able to get to services where and when they are needed. Accessibility can be seen in terms of *geographical distance* or of *travel times* from peoples' homes to mental health facilities. In other words, the principle of accessibility is one of the main reasons for developing decentralised care, and for offering community care and mobile teams.

Another type of accessibility means arranging services so that they do not mean long and bureaucratic delays in how long it takes for people to be assessed and

Table 4.2 Principles relevant to the mental health policies and mental health laws [21]

Principle	England 1999 [22]	Scotland 2003 [23]	United Nations 1992 [7]	WHO 2001 [24]	World Psychiatric Association 1996 [25]
(1) Participation	Involve service-users	Regard to past and present wishes of patient, … full patient participation		Consumer involvement … right to information and participation	Patient should be accepted as a partner by right in therapeutic process
(2) Therapeutic benefit to the individual patient	Effective care	Importance of providing maximum benefit to patient	Right to the best available mental health care. Every patient shall have the right to receive such health and social care as is appropriate to his r her health needs … in the best interest of the patient	Efficient treatment	Providing the best therapy available consistent with accepted scientific knowledge. Treatment must always be in the best interest of the patient
(3) Choice of acceptable treatments	Acceptable care and choice	Importance of providing ppropriate services to patient		Wide range of services	Allow the patient to make free and informed decisions
(4) Non-discrimination	Non-discriminatory	Have regard to encouragement of equal opportunities	These Principles shall be applied without discrimination of any kind	Equality and non-discrimination	Fair and equal treatment of the mentally ill. Discrimination by psychiatrists on the basis of ethnicity or culture, whether directly or by aiding others, is unethical

Table 4.2 (cont.)

Principle	England 1999 [22]	Scotland 2003 [23]	United Nations 1992 [7]	WHO 2001 [24]	World Psychiatric Association 1996 [25]
(5) Access	Accessible		Every patient shall have the right to be treated and cared for, as far as possible, in the community in which he or she lives	Local services	
(6) Safety	Promote safety		To protect the health or safety of the person concerned or of others, or otherwise to protect public safety, order, health or morals or the fundamental rights and freedoms of others.	Physical integrity of service-user	
(7) Autonomy and empowerment	Independence		Treatment ... directed towards preserving and enhancing personal autonomy.	Patient empowerment, autonomy	Provide the patient with relevant information so as to empower them
(8) Family involvement		Have regard to needs and circumstances of patient's carer		Partnership with families, involvement of local community	Psychiatrist should consult with the family

	Preserve dignity	Treated with humanity and respect for the inherent dignity of the human person		Psychiatrists to be guided primarily by the respect for patients and concern for their welfare and integrity … to safeguard the human dignity
(9) Dignity				
(10) Least restrictive form of care		Every patient shall have the right to be treated in the least restrictive environment	Have regard to minimum restriction of the freedom of the patient necessary	Therapeutic interventions that are least restrictive to the freedom of the patient
(11) Advocacy			Have regard to views of patient's named person, carer, guardian, welfare attorney	
(12) Capacity		The person whose capacity is at issue shall be entitled to be represented by a counsel		

Table 4.3 Principles guiding post-apartheid mental health law in South Africa

- The right to disclosure of information
- Rights to representation
- Protections over admissions to facilities
- Regulations against unfair discrimination,
- Rules regarding respect, consent, dignity and privacy
- Rights to be free from exploitations and abuse

Table 4.4 Values and principles guiding mental health policy in England [22]

Fundamental values that should be used to guide practical service developments.
  Service should:
- Show openness and honesty
- Demonstrate respect and offer courtesy
- Be allocated fairly and provided equitably
- Be proportional to needs
- Be open to learning and change

Fundamental principles, so that service-users can expect services to:
- Meaningfully involve users and their carers
- Deliver high quality treatment and care which is effective and acceptable
- Be non-discriminatory
- Be accessible: help when and where it is needed
- Promote user safety and that of their carers, staff and the wider public
- Offer choices which promote independence
- Be well co-ordinated between all staff and agencies
- Empower and support their staff
- Deliver continuity of care as long as needed
- Be accountable to the public, users and carers

treated. Third, access means that services are equally available to all those who need them, regardless of any *selective barriers* which reduce the uptake of services by particular groups (such as people with personality disorders), or for some sub-groups of the population (such as ethnic minorities). In addition, accessibility can refer to the openness of the service to service-users outside office hours, at night and at weekends, or to the public visibility of the service, as opposed to the remote institutions which were 'out-of-sight' and associated with shame.

There may be disadvantages associated with too much accessibility. For example, if services are too available, then service-users may have a low threshold to consult when in difficulty, may bypass primary care services where these exist, and may expect specialist attention when suffering from relatively minor conditions. Such contacts may divert time and resources away from more severely disabled service-users.

Table 4.5 Basic principles to be applied locally in developing services

Principle	Definition
(1) Autonomy	A patient characteristic consisting of the ability to make independent decisions and choices, despite the presence of symptoms or disabilities. Autonomy should be promoted by effective treatment and care.
(2) Continuity	The ability of the relevant services to offer interventions, at the patient or at the local level, (i) which refers to the coherence of interventions over a shorter time period, both within and between teams (*cross-sectional continuity*), or (ii) which are an uninterrupted series of contacts over a longer time period (*longitudinal continuity*)
(3) Effectiveness	At the local level we define *effectiveness* as 'the proven, intended benefits of services provided in real life situations'. At the patient level we define *effectiveness* as 'the proven, intended benefits of treatments provided in real life situations'.
(4) Accessibility	A service characteristic, experienced by users and their carers, which enables them to receive care where and when it is needed.
(5) Comprehensiveness	A service characteristic with two dimensions: (i) By *horizontal comprehensiveness* we mean how far a service extends across the whole range of severity of mental illnesses, and across a wide range of patient characteristics (gender, age, ethnic group, diagnosis). (ii) By *vertical comprehensiveness* we mean the availability of the basic components of care (out-patient and community care; day care; acute in-patient and longer-term residential care; interfaces with other services), and their use by prioritised groups of patients.
(6) Equity	The fair distribution of resources. The rationale used to prioritise between competing needs, and the methods used to calculate the allocation of resources, should be made explicit.
(7) Accountability	A function which consists of complex, dynamic relationships between mental health services and patients, their families and the wider public, who all have legitimate expectations of how the service should act responsibly.
(8) Co-ordination	A service characteristic which is manifested by coherent treatment plans for individual patients. Each plan should have clear goals and should include interventions which are needed and effective: no more and no less. By *cross-sectional co-ordination* we mean the co-ordination of information and services within an episode of care (both within and between services). By *longitudinal*

Table 4.5 (cont.)

Principle	Definition
	co-ordination we mean the inter-linkages between staff and between agencies over a longer period of treatment, often spanning several episodes.
(9) Efficiency	A service characteristic, which minimises the inputs needed to achieve a given level of outcomes, or which maximises the outcomes for a given level of inputs.

Table 4.6 Components of a comprehensive adult mental health care system

(1) Out-patient/ambulatory clinics
(2) Community mental health teams
(3) Acute in-patient care
(4) Long-term community-based residential care
(5) Employment and occupation

Comprehensiveness

In our view a comprehensive service is one that has all the elements of what can be described as a 'basic, comprehensive adult mental health care system', as summarised in Table 4.6 [28;29].

The degree of comprehensiveness of a service raises the key question: comprehensive for whom? Since mental health problems will affect about a third of the general adult population in any year, and since the capacity of the mental-health services, even in the most economically developed countries, means that they can provide a service usually to about 2% of the adult population, these services will *necessarily* be limited to only a minority of all people with mental illnesses. The question then becomes one of quality *or* quantity. Services which selectively treat first the more severely mentally ill, such as in Britain, will provide a relatively poor service for the majority of people with mental illness, many of whom will have anxiety-depression, and who will remain untreated if they are not recognised by primary care staff.

In some countries, such as Italy, it is not mandatory for referrals to specialist care to come from primary health care staff. More open access is therefore offered, for example by self-referral, in the name of a comprehensive service. The advantages of this system are that it may avoid delays and it may decrease the stigma associated with mental health service use, by making the service routinely available. The disadvantages are that since comprehensiveness is limited by the capacity of the service, it may develop in the 'wrong' direction. By this we mean that services given to people with lesser degrees of disability may replace those given to people with more severe forms of mental illness, more of whom may be left untreated.

In the latter case, this means that people with less disabling conditions are provided with care instead of those who are most disabled. This produces the following problems. *First*, people with these more severe disorders may not seek help, but may need a pattern of care which can include regular contact at home. *Second*, people with psychotic disorders, who accumulate in the lowest social class group, tend to have fewer choices than other service-users, may be ineffective advocates for their own interests and needs, and exercise relatively little political influence or financial market power. *Third*, over-provision of services can produce an 'induction effect' whereby service-users become used to receiving multiple types of service, whereas only one specific type of treatment may be justified on grounds of evidence. *Fourth*, setting comprehensiveness as a service goal, in an undefined way, can produce a gap for staff between expectations and clinical reality, which becomes a potent source of stress and burnout.

Continuity

Many people with enduring mental illness have an ongoing need for reliable sources of treatment and social support. The principle of continuity is poorly defined. It is possible to distinguish between longitudinal and cross-sectional dimensions of continuity of care. *Longitudinal continuity* refers to the ability of services to offer an uninterrupted series of contacts over a period of time [30]. This implies either continuity of the same staff group, even if the individual staff members change, or to provide some continuity across episodes of care, for example between in-patient and community treatment. An important second meaning of longitudinal continuity is to ensure a planned transfer of care between services when the service-user moves home.

Cross-sectional continuity includes continuity between different service-providers, which in practice means between different mental health teams or programmes. This refers especially to fragmented services. The second type of cross-sectional continuity applies within clinical teams, and refers to how far team members communicate with each other about their direct clinical work with service-users.

The advantages of placing an emphasis on continuity are that it is easier to give consistent treatment and care, and to avoid contradictory interventions, including those which the service-users' behaviour may provoke through the 'splitting' of staff teams. It may also be easier to predict relapses and remissions, and to intervene early. Further, an emphasis on continuity can develop stronger trusting relationships between staff and service-users, which is both desirable in itself and can be especially invaluable in crises [31].

Continuity can improve staff morale by keeping contact with the same group of service-users over a long enough time period to see improvement.

Communication can also help to provide a continuing service while individual members of staff are away on leave. Continuity of communication within the team also improves communication between the team and those outside, including the service-user's family, who will receive a more consistent message. This principle will also lead to a more unitary way of dealing with problems, including physical problems, and so encourages access to other specialists. Finally, continuity can also increase the possibility of helping service-users to solve practical problems, e.g. application for welfare benefits.

At the same time there are disadvantages from too much stress upon continuity. It can provide a rigid approach, which leaves the service-user feeling trapped. Continuity in practice can reduce choice for service-users, therapists and referrers. Continuity can also mean a slow rate of turnover of cases and this contains the possibility of producing staff disillusionment with longer-term service-users who deteriorate or who do not improve, and with those who are extremely demanding in the long term.

From the service-user's perspective, services organised to maximise continuity may limit access to a particular treatment if the case manager is not trained in that intervention. In other words, the trade-off can be between continuity and specialisation. In a system with home-treatment (crisis-resolution) teams [32], for example, they may be able to offer more intensive home support during periods of crisis, perhaps avoiding the need for hospital admission, but necessitating discontinuities, with frequent changes of staff contacts for service-users.

The greatest risk, however, is that a dependence on the service will be fostered, which encourages a chronically sick role, and which can inhibit moving towards recovery. For example, a high degree of continuity was offered in traditional mental hospitals, alongside a high degree of dependence. For these reasons we consider that a proper balance is needed to provide *variable continuity*. We would draw a parallel here with the use of medication. In the same way that we would sometimes encourage service-users to use intermittent medication, or to vary the dose within an agreed range, so we would suggest that the intensity with which continuity of care is provided should be varied so as to maintain and extend autonomy for each service-user.

Co-ordination

We can also distinguish between cross-sectional and longitudinal co-ordination. The first refers to the co-ordination of information and services within an episode of care. The latter refers to the links between staff and between agencies over a longer period of care. The communication necessary to ensure proper co-ordination can be informal or formal. In decentralised service systems, such as community mental health teams, more careful attention needs to be paid to clear lines of communication, since staff will less often see each other on a day-to-day basis than in a traditional hospital. This may mean that more formal systems of communication are needed, for example, daily morning handover meetings to inform all staff of clinical developments. The key role of the case manager is to provide co-ordination, both cross-sectional and longitudinal, indeed in Italian local Departments of Mental Health the role is referred to as 'coordinatore', and in England this role is called 'care co-ordinator'.

Guiding principles at the individual level

As we argued earlier in this book, in our view the main aim of mental health care is to achieve better *outcomes* for individuals with mental illness than would otherwise occur (cell 3C in the mental health matrix). By the same token, talk of principles is essentially meaningless unless it translates into better conditions, meaning better *processes* of care for individuals with mental illness. One important aspect is how far the basic human rights of mentally ill people are observed, as shown in Table 4.7.

A further way in which principles can be tested in practice is to assess how far people with mental illness are able to: (i) enjoy all the human rights available to the general population, and (ii) be treated with parity compared with people with physical disabilities [34]. In fact, stigma and discrimination stand fully in the way of all these rights and entitlements. The evidence here is compelling that in every country people with mental illness tend to be systematically excluded from normal social participation in terms of family life, childcare, work and social activities [35–37].

One example of a statement of principles relevant to the individual level is the 'Declaration of Madrid' of 1996. Developed over 20 years, after the Hawaii (1978) and Vienna (1983) guidelines, these are intended to be the minimal requirements for ethical standards of the psychiatric profession, applicable to a wide variety of cultural, legal, social and economic conditions. These principles were further revised in 1996 and the Madrid revision is summarised in Table 4.8 [25].

Table 4.7 Basic human rights to be observed for people with mental illness [33]

- Right to education
- Right to property
- Right to marry, to found a family, and to respect family life
- Right to vote
- Right to associate
- Right to work

Table 4.8 Summary of the Declaration of Madrid, 1996

(1) Psychiatry is concerned with the provision of the best treatment for mental disorders, with rehabilitation and the promotion of mental health.

(2) It is the duty of psychiatrists to keep abreast of scientific developments of the speciality.

(3) The patient should be accepted as a partner by right in the therapeutic process.

(4) When the patient is incapacitated and unable to exercise proper judgement because of a mental disorder, the psychiatrist should consult with the family, and, if appropriate, seek legal counsel to safeguard human dignity and the legal rights of the patient. Treatment must always be in the best interest of the patient.

(5) When psychiatrists are requested to assess a person, it is their duty to inform the person being assessed about the purpose of the intervention, about the use of the findings and about the possible repercussions of the assessment.

(6) Information obtained in the therapeutic relationship should be kept in confidence and used only for the purpose of improving the mental health of the patient.

(7) Research which is not conducted with the canons of science is unethical. Only individuals properly trained in research should undertake or direct it. Because psychiatric patients are particularly vulnerable research subjects, extra caution should be taken to safeguard their autonomy, as well as their mental and physical integrity.

Putting principles into practice

The principles described in this chapter can be used, not just for planning services, but also for clinical research, as shown in Table 4.9, adapted from Emmanuel *et al.* [38].

Principles may also be practically useful in considering which types of treatment are the most ethically acceptable. For example, in many countries it is seen to be best practice to use the least restrictive treatment in any given clinical situation to minimise coercion [39;40]. One aspect of coercion are laws or regulations which allow the compulsory treatment of people with mental illness outside hospital, and these provisions are variously called community treatment orders (CTO), or involuntary outpatient commitment [41;42]. If the principles of least restrictive alternative and effectiveness are given priority in a particular jurisdiction, then any review of CTOs will conclude there is no good evidence that CTOs are effective [43;44].

Our main point in this chapter is that neither the technical solutions of evidence-based medicine, nor the ideologically based views of individual stake-holder groups can be used alone to respond adequately to complex choices when planning and providing care. Rather, we suggest that a form of *trialogue* is necessary to inter-weave *ethical* considerations, a clear understanding of the *evidence* base, and the views and contributions of those with substantial *experience* in the mental health field.

Table 4.9 Requirements for making clinical research ethical

Ethical requirement	Key issues to consider
(1) Social or scientific value	Treatment/intervention that will improve health and increase knowledge
(2) Scientific validity	Use of accepted scientific principles and methods
(3) Fair subject selection	Stigmatised and vulnerable individuals are not targeted for risky research and the socially powerful not favoured for potentially beneficial research
(4) Favourable risk–benefit ratio	Minimisation of risks; enhancement of potential benefits
(5) Independent review	Review of the design of the research trial by individuals unaffiliated with the research
(6) Informed consent	Provision of information to subjects so that the individual can make a voluntary decision whether to enrol and continue to participate
(7) Respect of potential and enrolled subjects	Permitting withdrawal from the research – Protecting privacy – Informing of newly discovered risks and benefits – Informing of results of clinical research – Maintaining welfare of subjects

Table 4.10 Key stakeholders for involvement in discussing guiding principles

- Consumers/service-users
- Family members/carers
- Professionals
- Other service-provider groups, e.g. non-govermental organisations (NGOs)
- Policy-makers
- Advocacy groups
- Service-planners and commissioners

So far we have focussed upon *what* principles may be useful in planning and providing mental health services. Finally we would also like to briefly discuss *how* to decide which principles matter locally. It will usually be important to involve all the groups who have a real interest in such service changes ('stakeholders'), as shown in Table 4.10.

Stakeholder involvement is important for the positive reason that a more broadly based discussion is more likely to be carefully thought through and to lead to better solutions [45;46]. But there is also a less honourable reason: if a key group is excluded from these discussions, then it is likely that they will object to what the others decide! This may then slow down or even stop service developments. So, in our view, widespread participation in setting service principles is right in principle and right in practice!

Key points in this chapter

- We place ethics first as we consider that in health care there is no place for interventions which are technically effective, but which are unethical.
- It is better to make the ethical framework explicit early in a planning cycle.
- Important basic human rights for people with mental illness include rights to: education, property, marry, found a family and to respect family life, vote, associate and to work.
- Nine particular principles which may be applicable are: autonomy, continuity, effectiveness, accessibility, comprehensiveness, equity, accountability, co-ordination and efficiency (which may be called the three aces!).

REFERENCES

1. Downie RS and Calman KC. *Healthy Respect. Ethics in Healthcare*. London: Faber & Faber; 1987.
2. Beauchamp TL and Childress JF. *Principles of Biomedical Ethics*. Oxford: Oxford University Press; 1994.
3. Holm S. Not just autonomy. The principles of American biomedical ethics. *J. Med. Ethics* 1995; **21**: 332–338.
4. Baker D. Human rights for persons with disabilities. In Nagler M and Kemp EJ (Eds.). *Perspectives on Disability*. Palo Alto, CA: Health Markets Research; 1993. 483–494.
5. Amnesty International. *Ethical Codes and Declarations Relevant to the Health Professions*. London: Amnesty International; 2000.
6. Amnesty International. *Mental Illness, the Neglected Quarter: Summary Report*. Dublin: Amnesty International; 2003.
7. United Nations. *UN Principles for the Protection of Persons with Mental Illness and for the Improvement of Mental Health Care. Adopted by UN General Assembly Resolution 46/119 of 18 February 1992*. New York: United Nations; 1992.
8. United Nations. *Universal Declaration of Human Rights. Adopted and Proclaimed by the UN General Assembly Resolution 217A (III) of 10 December 1948*. New York: United Nations; 1948.
9. United Nations. *International Covenant on Civil and Political Rights. Adopted by the UN General Assembly Resolution 2200A (XXI) of 16 December 1966*. New York: United Nations (http://www.ohchr.org/english/countries/ratification/4.htm); 1966.
10. United Nations. *International Covenant on Economic, Social and Cultural Rights. Adopted by UN General Assembly Resolution 2200A (XXI) of 16 December 1966*. New York: United Nations; 1966.

11. United Nations. *Persons with Disabilities. General Comments Number 5 (Eleventh Session 1994).* UN Doc E/C 12/1994/13. UN Committee on Economic, Social and Cultural Rights. New York: United Nations; 1994.

12. World Health Organisation. *WHO Resource Book on Mental Health, Human Rights and Legislation.* Geneva: World Health Organisation; 2005.

13. Kingdon D, Jones R and Lonnqvist J. Protecting the human rights of people with mental disorder: new recommendations emerging from the Council of Europe. *Br. J. Psychiatry* 2004; **185**: 277–279.

14. Bindman J, Maingay S and Szmukler G. The Human Rights Act and mental health legislation. *Br. J. Psychiatry* 2003; **182**: 91–94.

15. Thornicroft G and Szmukler G. The draft Mental Health Bill in England: without principles. *Psychiatr. Bull.* 2005; **29**: 244–247.

16. Ministry of Health of Federative Republic of Brazil, PAHO, WHO. *The Brazilia Principles. Guiding Principles for the Development of Mental Health Care in the Americas.* Geneva: Ministry of Health of the Federative Republic of Brazil, PAHO and WHO; 2005.

17. Pan American Health Organization/WHO Regional Office for the Americas. *Declaration of Caracas (1990). Adopted on 14 November 1990 by the Regional Conference on the Restructuring of Psychiatric Care in Latin America, convened in Caracas, Venezuela.* Washington DC: Pan American Health Organization/WHO Regional Office for the Americas.; 1990.

18. World Health Organisation. *Mental Health Legislation and Human Rights.* Geneva: World Health Organisation; 2003.

19. World Health Organisation. *Mental Health Action Plan for Europe.* Copenhagen: World Health Organisation; 2005.

20. World Health Organisation. *Mental Health Declaration for Europe.* Copenhagen: World Health Organisation; 2005.

21. Thornicroft G and Szmukler G. The draft Mental Health Bill in England: without principles. *Psychiatr. Bull.* 2005; **29**: 244–247.

22. Department of Health. *National Service Framework for Mental Health. Modern Standards and Service Models.* London: Department of Health; 1999.

23. Scottish Executive. *Mental Health (Care and Treatment) (Scotland) Act.* Edinburgh: Scottish Executive; 2003.

24. World Health Organisation. World Health Report 2001. *Mental Health: New Understanding, New Hope.* Geneva: World Health Organization; 2001.

25. World Psychiatric Association. *Declaration of Madrid.* Geneva: World Psychiatric Association; 1996.

26. Thornicroft G and Tansella M. *The Mental Health Matrix: A Manual to Improve Services.* Cambridge: Cambridge University Press; 1999.

27. Thornicroft G and Tansella M. Translating ethical principles into outcome measures for mental health service research. *Psychol. Med.* 1999; **29**(4): 761–767.

28. Thornicroft G and Tansella M. The components of a modern mental health service: a pragmatic balance of community and hospital care. *Br. J. Psychiatry* 2004; **185**: 283–290.

29. Thornicroft G and Tansella M. *What Are the Arguments for Community-Based Mental Health Care?* Copenhagen: World Health Organisation (European Region) Health Evidence Network; 2003.

30. Johnson S, Prosser D, Bindman J and Szmukler G. Continuity of care for the severely mentally ill: concepts and measures. *Soc. Psychiatry Psychiatr. Epidemiol.* 1997; **32** (3): 137–142.

31. Henderson C, Flood C, Leese M, *et al.* Effect of joint crisis plans on use of compulsory treatment in psychiatry: single blind randomised controlled trial. *BMJ* 2004; **329**(7458): 136–138.

32. Johnson S, Needle J, Bindman J and Thornicroft G. *Crisis Resolution and Home Treatment in Mental Health.* Cambridge: Cambridge University Press; 2008.

33. Bartlett P, Lewis O and Thorold O. *Mental Disability and the European Convention on Human Rights.* Leiden: Martinus Nijhoff; 2006.

34. Thornicroft G. *Actions Speak Louder: Tackling Discrimination against People with Mental Illness.* London: Mental Health Foundation; 2006.

35. Corrigan P. *On the Stigma of Mental Illness.* Washington, DC: American Psychological Association; 2005.

36. Thornicroft G. *Shunned: Discrimination against People with Mental Illness.* Oxford: Oxford University Press; 2006.

37. Sartorius N and Schulze H. *Reducing the Stigma of Mental Illness. A Report from a Global Programme of the World Psychiatric Association.* Cambridge: Cambridge University Press; 2005.

38. Emmanuel EJ, Wendler D and Gradi C. What makes clinical research ethical? *JAMA* 2000; (283): 2701–2711.

39. Appelbaum P and Szmukler G. Treatment pressures, coercion and compulsion. In Thornicroft G and Szmukler G (Eds.). *Textbook of Community Psychiatry.* Oxford: Oxford University Press; 2001.

40. Bindman J, Reid Y, Szmukler G, *et al.* Perceived coercion at admission to psychiatric hospital and engagement with follow-up – a cohort study. *Soc. Psychiatry Psychiatr. Epidemiol.* 2005; **40**(2): 160–166.

41. Kisely S and Campbell LA. Does compulsory or supervised community treatment reduce 'revolving door' care?: Legislation is inconsistent with recent evidence. *Br. J. Psychiatry* 2007; **191**: 373–374.

42. Kisely S, Campbell LA, Scott A, Preston NJ and Xiao J. Randomized and non-randomized evidence for the effect of compulsory community and involuntary out-patient treatment on health service use: systematic review and meta-analysis. *Psychol. Med.* 2007; **37**(1): 3–14.

43. Kisely S, Campbell L and Preston N. Compulsory community and involuntary outpatient treatment for people with severe mental disorders. *Cochrane Database Syst. Rev.* 2005; **3**: CD004408.

44. Ridgely MS, Borum R and Petrila J. *The Effectiveness of Involuntary Outpatient Treatment.* Santa Monica: RAND Corporation; 2001.

45. Pescosolido BA, Wright ER and Kikuzawa S. 'Stakeholder' attitudes over time toward the closing of a state hospital. *J. Behav. Health Serv. Res.* 1999; **26**(3): 318–328.

46. Griffiths KM, Jorm AF, Christensen H, Medway J and Dear KB. Research priorities in mental health, Part 2: an evaluation of the current research effort against stake-holders' priorities. *Aust. N. Z. J. Psychiatry* 2002; **36**(3): 327–339.

5

The evidence base for mental health care

The aim of this chapter is to describe a stepwise approach to identifying the available evidence for better mental health care. We shall first describe the background epidemiological information which can support service planning. Next we shall discuss how local service utilisation data contribute to the evidence base that can inform planning. Finally we shall consider the different components of a comprehensive mental health system of care, according to the available resources.

At the outset it is important to appreciate that such planning decisions need to take place in the context of a broad understanding of the health and social care needs of the whole population in question. Further, in our view there is no 'best' pattern of services, rather a balance of service components, which have a reasonable 'degree-of-fit' to local circumstances. Similarly, in any local setting there exists no 'correct' scale of provision, only estimates based on the best available data. In other words we encourage you to find local solutions to local challenges.

Epidemiologically based measures of local prevalence rates

It is usually helpful to have a clear view of the mental health needs of the population for whom services are being provided. Table 5.1 indicates a series of steps to find the best available information on population prevalence rates.

As Table 5.1 shows, we consider that the best possible information would be local epidemiological data on the occurrence of mental disorders, using a standard system of classification, alongside a measure of the needs for treatment among the prevalent cases identified [1]. Since these assessments are expensive and time consuming, most sites will not have access to such recent local data. If the data in step (1) are not available then we suggest that country/regional epidemiological data (2) are used instead, and are then weighted for local socio-demographic characteristics. But if such larger-scale prevalence data are not available, then a third option is to use international rates from 'comparison'

Table 5.1 Ways to estimate mental illness prevalence in the local population

---

(1) Actual local epidemiological data on psychiatric morbidity and disability for the particular area by age, sex, ethnicity, social status, and degree of urbanicity

(if not available)
↓

(2) Country/regional epidemiological data weighted for local socio-demographic characteristics

(if not available)
↓

(3) International data from 'comparable' countries or regions, adjusted for local socio-demographic characteristics

(If 1, 2, 3 not sufficient)
↓

(4) Best estimates and expert synthesis and interpretation based on other sources of local information and opinions (e.g. extent of non-health-service provision, family support, local traditions, or migration)

---

countries or regions, again weighted for local socio-demographic characteristics (3). The results in this case will be less accurate because they are based on the additional assumption that the data can be transferred between countries.

In some cases, none of the data described in steps (1)–(3) will be available, and then the next option (4) is to use a number of experts, some of whom may be from the local area, to produce a consensus statement on the local rates and characteristics of people with mental illness. Such a data synthesis can be based on the best available views, taking into account local factors (e.g. levels of non-health-service provision, family support, traditions, degree of affluence or migration).

Actual service provision data as information for planning

Another dimension in using evidence to support service planning and provision is to consider what services are actually provided on the ground. Table 5.2 shows some of the key points that need to be considered here. For example, it is important to be clear about which types of care are provided through the first level of general health services (primary care), which are provided by specialist mental health care (secondary care) and which by sub-specialist teams (tertiary). The assessment of actual service provision can take place at two levels: (i) the contacts and services that are provided within each clinical unit or team (service components), and (ii) how far these constituent parts work well together as a whole service system. This second question requires information about, for example, the flows of service users between different service components.

Table 5.2 Service provision data

- *Define categories* of service components for primary, secondary and tertiary levels of care (see general adult mental-health care model in Section 5.4)
- *Quantify the capacities* of the service components (e.g. number of beds – in hospital or in alternative settings – or number of cases treated by a home treatment team at any one time)
- *Assess the quality of care* of the service sites (for example as assessed by a quality inspectorate or by service-users/carers)
- *Collect quantitative and qualitative* information on staff (including morale and sickness rates)
- *Evaluate the degree of integration and co-ordination* of components into a whole-service system

This whole-system approach will also address the question of whether any categories of people with mental illness are underserved or even completely untreated by any part of the care system. How far the whole system approach can be applied in practice depends in large part upon the way in which health care is funded and organised in each particular area. The whole-system view is more readily usable in state/national health services which have a unified system for commissioning or providing care. Methods have been developed to guide the description of mental health care in a structured way. For example, the International Classification of Mental Health Care (WHO-ICMHC) [2] is one way to do this. More recently the European Service Mapping Schedule has been developed for the same purpose [3].

Using service utilisation data

Having set the scene by describing the service landscape, it is then possible to assess the dynamic working of these service components. Data on local service use may refer either to clinical events or to individuals, and can be described under four headings:

(1) *Event-based information for a given service component*, (e.g. annual number, or rate, of admissions).

(2) *Individual-based information for a particular service component* (e.g. annual number, or rate, of separate individuals who receive out-patient services).

(3) *Individual-based information on episodes of illness*, from onset to recovery (e.g. annual number, or rate, of episodes of depression treated by a given service).

(4) *Individual-based information on episodes of care* (e.g. annual number, or rate, of episodes of treatment for anorexia).

Table 5.3 Examples of service utilisation data

- 'Event-based' data on clinical contacts by levels of care (in-patient, out-patient etc.), number of events and rates per 10 000 population per year
- Individual-based data on both clinical contacts (as above) and on treatment episodes across different levels of care per year
- Data on outcomes and costs of different clinical contacts (disaggregated for sub-groups of patients) with which to establish substitutability and complementarity of service components in terms of cost-effectiveness

A profile of actual service use in any local area can be made, for example, using the categories shown in Table 5.3 (see Section 10.3 in our previous book for a more detailed discussion [4]). How many people receive treatment each year in each part of the service? What is the flow of people between these constituent parts of the system? Can particular blocks or barriers be identified which prevent people receiving care in the right part of the treatment system?

Predictions of service utilisation can also be the basis of allocating financial resources to different areas. To be useful such models need to be simple and based upon easily available data. For example, census data have been used in England and Italy to predict psychiatric hospital admission rates, and have been shown to be able to predict about 70% of the variation in such rates within each country. These approaches combine such factors as material poverty (e.g. from car ownership rates), education-employment, relational network, age profile (% of elderly living alone) or demographic factors (e.g. ethnicity) [5–7].

There are important connections between the supply of care in each local area and the types of demand made of them. *First*, where psychiatric beds are available then they are filled, whatever the quantity of provision [8]. *Second*, the categories of service used are usually entirely governed by the types of service available locally. If, for example, home-treatment services are not provided in a given area, then the options available to staff when assessing a patient in crisis are normally restricted to in-patient or day-hospital admission. In this way supply, in turn, also shapes demand in that the family of a patient in crisis may demand an admission, since in their experience this is the only option which can help. *Third*, the use of the services provided depends to a large extent upon the system turnover, or, in the case of beds, for example, the average length of stay. In other words, both structural and dynamic aspects need to be considered simultaneously.

Evidence for a balance of hospital and community care

If we want to plan on the basis of evidence, we need now to move to more direct and practical questions. For the particular area being considered, which services are being provided reasonably well, and which need to be introduced or strengthened? To answer this we need to know what resources are available for mental health care, and also we need to have an overall scheme which allows us to know which service components are necessary for each level of available resources. This scheme therefore supports decisions about what are higher or lower priorities when developing mental health care.

In this section we shall argue for a 'stepped-care' model for adult mental health services and we shall present the evidence for this approach. From a thorough review of the scientific literature, especially focussing upon 'effectiveness' studies [9], we will discuss particular service components, and present the findings in terms of service models which are suitable for areas with low, medium and high levels of resources [10], as discussed in the WHO World Health Report [11]. Both the stepped-care scheme and the three types of resource level are clearly over-simplified, and are solely intended to make complex realities more manageable.

Table 5.4 indicates that areas with low level of resources (Column 1) can only afford to provide most or all of their mental health care in primary health care settings, delivered by primary-care staff. The very limited specialist back-up can then offer: training, consultation for complex cases, and in-patient assessment and treatment for cases which cannot be managed in primary care [12;13]. Some low-resource countries may in fact be in a pre-asylum stage [14], in which apparent community care in fact represents widespread neglect of mentally ill people. Where asylums do exist, policy-makers face difficult choices about whether to upgrade the quality of care they offer [14], or to convert the resources of the larger hospitals into decentralised services instead [15].

We have deliberately separated the types of care into these three schemes because the differences in mental health care which are possible in low and high resource areas (both between and within countries) are vast. In Europe, for example, there are between 5.5 and 20.0 psychiatrists per 100 000 population, whereas the figure is 0.5/100 000 in African countries [14]; the average number of psychiatric beds is 87 per 100 000 population in the European region, and 3.4 in Africa [15], and about 5–10% of the total health budget is spent on mental health in Europe [16], whereas in the African continent, 80% of countries spend less than 1% of their limited total health budget on mental health. Relevant comparative data is available from the WHO Project Atlas website [http://www.who.int/mental_health] [17].

Areas (countries or regions) with a medium level of resources may first establish the service components shown in Column 2, and later, as resources allow, choose to add some of the wider range of more highly specialised services indicated in Column 3. The choice of which of these more specialised services to develop first depends upon local factors including: services traditions and specific circumstances, consumer, carer and staff preferences, existing services strengths and weaknesses, and the way in which evidence is interpreted and used.

Table 5.4 Mental health service components in low, medium and high levels of resource areas: a stepped-care model

1. Low level of resource areas	2. Medium level of resource areas	3. High level of resource areas
(Step A) Primary mental-health care with specialist back-up	(Step A) Primary mental-health care with specialist back-up *and* (Step B) General adult mental-health care	(Step A) Primary mental-health care with specialist back-up *and* (Step B) General adult mental-health care *and* (Step C) Highly specialised mental-health care
Screening and assessment by primary-care staff Talking treatments including counselling and advice Pharmacological treatment Liaison and training with mental-health specialist staff, when available Limited specialist back-up available for: – training – consultation for complex cases – in-patient assessment and treatment for cases which cannot be managed in primary care, for example in general hospitals	1 Out-patient/ambulatory clinics	1 Specialised clinics for specific disorders or patient groups including: – eating disorders – dual diagnosis – treatment-resistant affective disorders – adolescent services
	2 Community mental-health teams	2 Specialised community mental-health teams including: – early interventions teams – assertive community treatment
	3 Acute in-patient care	3 Alternatives to acute hospital admission including: – home treatment / crisis resolution teams – crisis / respite houses – acute day hospitals
	4 Long-term community-based residential care	4 Alternative types of long-stay community residential care including: – intensive 24 hours staffed residential provision – less intensively staffed accommodation – independent accommodation
	5 Rehabilitation, occupation and work	5 Alternative forms of rehabilitation, occupation and work: – sheltered workshops – supervised work placements – co-operative work schemes – self-help and user groups – club houses/transitional employment programmes – vocational rehabilitation – individual placement and support

This stepped-care model also indicates that the forms of care relevant and affordable to areas with a high level of resources will add elements from Column 3 in addition to the components in Columns 1 and 2, which will usually already be present. The model is therefore *additive* and *sequential* in that new resources allow extra levels of service to be provided over time, in terms of mixtures of the components within each step, when the provision of the components in each previous step is complete.

Primary mental-health care with specialist back-up

Well-defined psychological problems are common in general health care and primary health care settings in every country, and cause disability which is usually in proportion to the number of symptoms present [18]. In areas with a low level of resources (Column 1) the large majority of cases of mental disorders should be recognised and treated within primary health care [19]. The WHO has shown that the integration of essential mental health treatments within primary health care in these countries is feasible [11].

General adult mental health care

This refers to a range of service components in areas that can afford more than a primary mental health care system. However, the recognition and treatment of the majority of people with mental illnesses, especially depression and anxiety-related disorders, remains a task which falls to primary care. The elements necessary in such a basic form of a comprehensive mental health service can be called 'general adult mental health care' and this is an amalgam of the following five core components:

(1) Out-patient/ambulatory clinics

These vary according to: whether people can self-refer or need to be referred by other agencies, such as primary care; whether there are fixed appointment times or open access assessments; whether doctors alone or other disciplines also provide clinical contact; whether direct or indirect payment is made; methods to enhance attendance rates; how to respond to non-attenders; and the frequency and duration of clinical contacts.

There is surprisingly little evidence on all of these key characteristics of out-patient care [20], but there is a strong clinical consensus in many countries that such clinics are a relatively efficient way to organise the provision of assessment and treatment, providing that the clinic sites are accessible to local populations. Nevertheless these clinics are simply methods of arranging clinical contact between staff and patients, and so the key issue is the *content* of the clinical interventions, namely to deliver treatments which are known to be evidence-based [21–23].

(2) Community mental health teams (CMHTs)

Community mental health teams are the basic building block for community mental health services. The simplest model of provision of community care is for generic (non-specialised) CMHTs to provide the full range of interventions (including the contributions of psychiatrists, community psychiatric nurses, social workers, psychologists and occupational therapists), usually prioritising adults with severe mental illness, for a local defined geographical catchment area [24;25]. A series of studies and systematic reviews, comparing CMHTs with a variety of hospital-based services, suggests that there are clear benefits to the introduction of generic community-based multi-disciplinary teams: they can improve engagement with services, increase user satisfaction, increase met needs and improve adherence to treatment, although they do not improve symptoms or social function [26–31]. In addition, continuity of care and service flexibility have been shown to be more developed where a CMHT model is in place [32].

Case management is a method of *delivering* care rather than being a clinical intervention in its own right, and at this stage the evidence suggests that it can most usefully be implemented within the context of CMHTs [33]. It is a style of working which has been described as the 'co-ordination, integration and allocation of individualised care within limited resources' [34]. There is now considerable literature to show that case management can be moderately effective in improving continuity of care, quality of life and patient satisfaction, but there is conflicting evidence on whether it has any impact on the use of in-patient services [35–39]. Case management needs to be carefully distinguished from the much more specific and more intensive *assertive community treatment* (see below).

(3) Acute in-patient care

There is no evidence that a balanced system of mental health care can be provided without acute beds. Some services (such as home-treatment teams, crisis house and acute day-hospital care, see below) may be able to offer realistic alternative care for some voluntary patients [40;41]. Nevertheless those who need urgent medical assessment, or those with severe and co-morbid medical and psychiatric conditions, severe psychiatric relapse and behavioural disturbance, high levels of suicidality or assaultiveness, acute neuro-psychiatric conditions, or elderly people with concomitant severe physical disorders, will usually require high intensity immediate support in acute in-patient hospital units.

There is a relatively weak evidence base on many aspects of in-patient care, and most studies are descriptive accounts [42]. There are few systematic reviews in this field, one of which found that there were no differences in outcomes between routine admissions and planned short hospital stays [43]. More generally, although there is a consensus that acute in-patient units are necessary, the number of beds required is highly contingent upon which other services exist locally and upon local social and cultural characteristics [4]. Acute in-patient care commonly absorbs most of the mental health budget [44], therefore minimising the use of bed-days, for example by reducing the average length of stay, may be an important goal, if the resources released in this way can be used for other service components. A related policy issue concerns how to provide acute beds in a humane and less institutionalised way that is acceptable to patients, for example in general hospital units [45;46].

(4) Long-term community-based residential care

It is important to know whether people with severe and long-term disabilities should still be cared for in larger, traditional institutions, or be transferred to long-term community-based residential care. The evidence here, for medium- and high-resource level areas, is clear. When deinstitutionalisation is carefully carried out, for those who have previously received long-term in-patient care for many years, then the outcomes are more favourable for most people who are discharged to community care [47–49]. The TAPS study in London [50], for example, completed a five-year follow-up on over 95% of 670 discharged long-stay non-demented people and found:

- Two thirds of the people were still living in their new residence.
- There was no increase in the death rate or the suicide rate.
- Very few people became homeless, and none were lost to follow up in staffed homes.
- Over one third were briefly readmitted, and at follow-up 10% of the sample were in hospital.
- Quality of life was greatly improved by the move to the community.
- There was little difference between total hospital and total community costs.
- Community care is therefore more cost-effective than long-stay hospital care.

Nevertheless, there is less evidence available on the treatment and care needs of the never institutionalised group of long-term patients [51], and so careful local assessments of the needs of this population are especially important. The range and capacity of community residential long-term care that will be needed in any particular area is also highly dependent upon which other services are available locally, and upon social and cultural factors, such as the amount of family care which is provided [52].

(5) Rehabilitation, occupation and work

Rates of unemployment among people with mental disorders are usually much higher than in the general population [53;54], and are also higher than among people with severe physical disabilities [55]. Traditional methods of occupation and day care have been day centres or a variety of psychiatric rehabilitation centres [56;57]. There is little hard evidence about these models of day care, and a recent review of over 300 papers, for example, found no relevant randomised controlled trials. Non-randomised studies have given conflicting results and for areas with medium levels of resources it is reasonable at this stage to make pragmatic decisions about the provision of rehabilitation, occupation and work services if the more highly specialised and evidence-based options discussed below are not affordable [58;59].

Highly specialised mental health services

The stepped-care model suggests that areas with high levels of resources may already provide all or most of the service components in Steps A and B, and are then able to offer additional components from the options shown in Step C in Table 5.4.

(1) Out-patient/ambulatory clinics

Highly specialised out-patient facilities for particular disorders or patient groups are common in many high-resource areas and may include, for example, services dedicated to: people with eating disorders; people with dual diagnosis (psychotic disorders and substance abuse); cases of treatment-resistant affective or psychotic disorders; those requiring specialised forms of psychotherapy; mentally disordered offenders; mentally ill mothers and their babies; and those with other specific disorders (such as post-traumatic stress disorder). Local decisions about whether to establish such highly specialised clinics will depend upon several factors, including their relative priority in relation to the other highly specialised services described below, identified services gaps and the financial opportunities available.

(2) Community mental health teams

These are by far the most researched of all the components of balanced care, and most randomised controlled trials and systematic reviews in this field refer to such teams [37]. Two types of highly specialised community mental health team have been particularly well developed as adjuncts to generic CMHTs: assertive community treatment (ACT) teams and early intervention (EI) teams.

Assertive community treatment teams

These provide a form of highly specialised mobile outreach treatment for people with more disabling mental disorders, and have been clearly character-ised [60–63]. There is now strong evidence that ACT can produce the following advantages in high level of resource areas: (i) reduce admissions to hospital and the use of acute beds; (ii) improve accommodation status and occupation and (iii) increase service-user satisfaction. ACT has not been shown to produce improvements in mental state or social behaviour. ACT can reduce the cost of in-patient services, but does not change the overall costs of care [64–66]. Nevertheless, it is not known how far ACT is cross-culturally relevant and, indeed, there is evidence that ACT may be less effective where usual services already offer high levels of continuity of care, for example in the UK, than in settings where the treatment as the usual control condition may offer little to people with severe mental illnesses [67–69].

Early intervention teams

There has been considerable interest in recent years in the prompt identi-fication and treatment of first or early episode cases of psychosis. Much of this research has focussed upon the time between first clear onset of symp-toms and the beginning of treatment, referred to as the 'duration of untreated psychosis' (DUP), while other studies have placed more emphasis upon providing family interventions when a young person's psychosis is first identified [70;71]. There is now emerging evidence that longer DUP is a predictor of worse outcome for psychosis; in other words, if patients wait a long time after developing a psychotic condition before they receive treat-ment, then they may take longer to recover and have a less favourable long-term prognosis.

Few controlled trials have been published of such interventions [72;73], and a Cochrane systematic review [74] has concluded that there are 'insufficient trials to draw any definitive conclusions, … the substantial international interest in early intervention offers an opportunity to make major positive changes in psychiatric practice, but this opportunity may be missed without a concerted international programme of research to address key unanswered questions'. It is therefore currently premature to judge whether specialised early intervention teams should be seen as a priority [75–80].

(3) Alternatives to acute in-patient care

In recent years three main alternatives to acute in-patient care have been developed: acute day hospitals, crisis houses and home treatment/crisis reso-lution teams. *Acute day hospitals* are facilities which offer programmes of day treatment for those with acute and severe psychiatric problems, as an alter-native to admission to in-patient units. A recent systematic review of nine randomised controlled trials has established that acute day-hospital care is suitable for about 30% of people who would otherwise be admitted to hospital, and offers advantages in terms of faster improvement and lower cost. It is reasonable to conclude that acute day-hospital care is an effective option when demand for in-patient beds is high [59;81].

Crisis houses are houses in community settings which are staffed by trained mental health professionals and offer admission for some people who would otherwise be admitted to hospital. A wide variety of respite houses, havens and refuges have been developed, but crisis house is used here to mean facilities which are alternatives to non-compulsory hospital admission. The little available research evidence suggests that they are very acceptable to their residents [42;82–84], may be able to offer an alternative to hospital admission for about a quarter of otherwise admitted patients, and may be more cost-effective than hospital admission [83;85;86]. Nevertheless there is emerging evidence that female patients, in particular, prefer non-hospital alternatives (such as single-sex crisis houses) to acute in-patient treatment, and this may reflect the lack of perceived safety in those settings [87].

Home-treatment/crisis-resolution teams are mobile community mental health teams offering assessment for people in psychiatric crises and providing intensive treatment and care at home. The key active ingredients appear to be regular home visits, and the combined provision of health and social care [88].

A Cochrane systematic review [88] found that most of the research evidence is from the USA or the UK, and concluded that home-treatment teams reduce days spent in hospital, especially if the teams make regular home visits and have responsibility for both health and social care [89]. Indeed a national study in England between 1998 and 2003 found that hospital admissions were reduced by 10% in areas which had crisis-resolution teams, and by 23% where these teams offered a 24 hour on-call system [90].

Crisis plans and advance directives: a Joint Crisis Plan (JCP) aims to empower the holder and to facilitate early detection and treatment of relapse [91]. It is developed by a patient together with mental health staff. Held by the patient, it contains his or her choice of information, which can include an advance agreement for treatment preferences for any future emergency, when he or she might be too unwell to express coherent views. The JCP format was developed after consultation with national user-groups, interviews with organisations and individuals using crisis cards [92], and detailed development work with service-users in South London. The results of the pilot study [93] showed that (at 6–12 month follow-up) 57% of participating patients felt more involved in their care, 60% felt more positive about their situation, 51% felt more in control of their mental health problem and 41% were more likely to continue treatment [1]. The JCP may have direct and indirect effects: family doctors and carers may be able to react earlier to a relapse, while emergency department staff may make better decisions when informed by the JCP. Negotiating the content may clarify treatment issues and build consensus between patients and staff, potentially reducing future compulsion in treatment and care. Recent research has shown that JCPs are able to halve the rates of compulsory treatment in hospital [94], and are cost-effective [95].

(4) Alternative types of long-stay community residential care

These are usually replacements for long-stay wards in psychiatric institutions [49;96;97]. Three categories of such residential care can be identified: (i) *24 hour staffed residential care* (high-staffed hostels, residential care homes or nursing homes, depending on whether the staff have professional qualifications); (ii) *day-staffed residential places* (hostels or residential homes which are staffed during the day) and (iii) *lower supported accommodation* (minimally supported hostels or residential homes with visiting staff). There is limited evidence on the cost-effectiveness of these types of residential care, and no completed systematic reviews [98]. It is therefore reasonable for policy-makers to decide upon the need for such services with local stakeholders [1;57;99;100].

(5) Alternative forms of rehabilitation, occupation and work

Although vocational rehabilitation has been offered in various forms to people with severe mental illnesses for over a century, its role has weakened because of discouraging results, financial disincentives to work and pessimism about outcomes for these patients [101–105]. However, recent alternative forms of occupation and vocational rehabilitation have again raised employment as an outcome priority. Consumer and carer advocacy groups have set work and occupation as one of their highest priorities, to enhance both functional status and quality of life [106–108].

There are recent indications that it is possible to improve vocational and psychosocial outcomes with supported employment models, which emphasise rapid placement in competitive jobs and support from employment specialists [109]. This individual placement and support (IPS) model emphasises competitive employment in integrated work settings with follow-up support [110]. Studies of IPS programmes have been encouraging in terms of increased rates of competitive employment [59;111;112].

This overview makes clear that there is no compelling argument and no scientific evidence favouring the use of hospital services alone. On the other hand, there is also no evidence that community services alone can provide satisfactory and comprehensive care. Both the evidence available so far, and accumulated clinical experience, therefore support a *balanced approach*, which includes both elements of hospital and community care [113].

The material resources available will severely constrain how this approach is applied in practice. In low-resource areas it may be unrealistic to invest in any of the components described here as general adult mental health care (Step B), and the focus will need to be upon primary mental health care, where the main role for the relatively few specialist mental health staff is to support primary-care staff (Step A, Column 1 in Table 5.4).

Areas which can afford a more highly specialised model of care may first consolidate what is described here as general adult mental health care (Step B), with the capacity of each service component decided as a balance between the known local needs [1], the resources available and the priorities of local stake-holders. In general, as mental health systems develop away from an asylum-based model, so the proportion of the total budget spent on the large institutions usually gradually decreases. In other words, new services outside hospital can only be provided by using extra resources (which is uncommon), or by using the resources which are transferred out from the hospital sites and staff (which is the more usual case). Interestingly, the evidence from cost-effectiveness studies, where they have been applied in relation to deinstitutionalisation and the provision of community mental health teams, is that the quality of care is closely related to the expenditure upon services, and overall community-based models of care are largely equivalent in cost to the services which they replace.

Over time, and as resources allow, each of the components of the general adult model can be complemented by additional and differentiated options, described here as differentiated/specialised mental services (Step C). Notably, the evidence base for these more recent and innovative forms of care is stronger than for any of the service components in Steps A or B, described above in relation to lower resource countries, and indeed very few high-quality scientific studies have been carried out in low-income countries [114;115]. Therefore the relevance of most published research in this field to less economically developed countries may be low. This schema therefore places the evidence of effective services within the appropriate resource context. Resource here refers, not only to the monetary investments made, but also to the available numbers of staff, their levels of experience and expertise, their therapeutic orientation and the contributions available from the wider social and family networks [19].

Two important implications arise from this approach. First, the stepped care model suggests that there should be a degree of co-ordination between service components, and, in particular, between the provision of primary and specialist (both general adult and highly specialised) care. We recognise that such planning mechanisms may be weak in some areas. Second, this model implies that the training of mental health staff should be fit for purpose according to the service stage reached (A, B or C), and the level of resources in the area (high, medium or low). In practice it is likely that, in any particular area, some, but not all, of the service components described here will be present, and that such identified gaps may inform local care planning.

Key points in this chapter

- Low income countries most often rely upon community-based and primary mental health care with very limited specialist back-up.
- Medium-resources countries are able to supplement this with the five categories of general adult mental health care: (1) out-patient/ambulatory clinics; (2) community mental health teams; (3) acute in-patient care; (4) long-term community-based residential care and (5) rehabilitation, occupation and work.
- High-resources countries can add to these two levels additional services (highly specialised mental health care in each of these five categories).
- The evidence available, and accumulated clinical experience, support a *balanced approach*, which includes both elements of community care with a limited provision of hospital care.
- New services outside hospital can only be provided by using extra resources (which is uncommon), or by using resources which are transferred out from hospitals (which is more usual).

REFERENCES

1. Thornicroft G. *Measuring Mental Health Needs*, 2nd edn. London: Royal College of Psychiatrists, Gaskell; 2001.
2. World Health Organisation. *International Classification of Mental Health Care*, 2nd edn. Copenhagen: WHO Regional Office for Europe and WHO Collaborating Centre for Research and Training in Mental Health, University of Groningen; 1990.
3. Johnson S and Kuhlmann R. The European Service Mapping Schedule (ESMS): development of an instrument for the description and classification of mental health services. *Acta Psychiatr. Scand. Suppl.* 2000; **405**: 14–23.
4. Thornicroft G and Tansella M. *The Mental Health Matrix: A Manual to Improve Services*. Cambridge: Cambridge University Press; 1999.
5. Thornicroft G. Social deprivation and rates of treated mental disorder. Developing statistical models to predict psychiatric service utilisation. *Br. J. Psychiatry* 1991; **158**: 475–484.
6. Tello JE, Jones J, Bonizzato P, *et al.* A census-based socio-economic status (SES) index as a tool to examine the relationship between mental health services use and deprivation. *Soc. Sci. Med.* 2005; **61**(10): 2096–2105.
7. Glover GR, Leese M and McCrone P. More severe mental illness is more concentrated in deprived areas. *Br. J. Psychiatry* 1999; **175**: 544–548.

8. Hansson L. Utilization of psychiatric inpatient care. A study of changes related to the introduction of a sectorized care organization. *Acta Psychiatr. Scand.* 1989; **79** (6): 571–578.

9. Tansella M, Thornicroft G, Barbui C, Cipriani A and Saraceno B. Seven criteria to improve effectiveness trials in psychiatry. *Psychol. Med.* 2006; **36**(5): 711–720.

10. Thornicroft G and Tansella M. Components of a modern mental health service: a pragmatic balance of community and hospital care: overview of systematic evidence. *Br. J. Psychiatry* 2004; **185**: 283–290.

11. World Health Organisation. World Health Report 2001. *Mental Health: New Understanding, New Hope.* Geneva: World Health Organization; 2001.

12. Mubbashar M. Mental health services in rural Pakistan. In Tansella M and Thornicroft G (Eds.). *Common Mental Disorders in Primary Care.* London: Routledge; 1999: 67–80.

13. Saxena S and Maulik P. Mental health services in low and middle income countries: an overview. *Curr. Opin. Psychiatry* 2003; **16**: 437–442.

14. Njenga F. Challenges of balanced care in Africa. *World Psychiatry* 2002; **1**: 96–98.

15. Alem A. Community-based vs. hospital-based mental health care: the case of Africa. *World Psychiatry* 2002; **1**: 99–100.

16. Becker T and Vazquez-Barquero JL. The European perspective of psychiatric reform. *Acta. Psychiatr. Scand. Suppl.* 2001;(410): 8–14.

17. World Bank. World Development Report 2002. *Building Institutions for Markets.* Washington DC: World Bank; 2002.

18. Ormel J, Von Korff M, Ustun B, Pini S and Korten A. Common mental disorders and disability across cultures. Results from the WHO Collaborative Study on Psychological Problems in General Health Care. *JAMA* 1994; **272**: 1741–1748.

19. Desjarlais R, Eisenberg L, Good B and Kleinman A. *World Mental Health. Problems and Priorities in Low Income Countries.* Oxford: Oxford University Press; 1995.

20. Becker T. Out-patient psychiatric services. In Thornicroft G and Szmukler G (Eds.). *Textbook of Community Psychiatry.* Oxford: Oxford University Press; 2001: 277–282.

21. Nathan P and Gorman J. *A Guide to Treatments That Work*, 2nd edn. Oxford: Oxford University Press; 2002.

22. Roth A and Fonagy P. *What Works for Whom? A Critical Review of Psychotherapy Research.* New York: Guildford Press; 1996.

23. BMJ Books. *Clinical Evidence*, Vol. 9 edn. London: BMJ Books; 2003.

24. Thornicroft G, Becker T, Holloway F, *et al.* Community mental health teams: evidence or belief? *Br. J. Psychiatry* 1999; **175**: 508–513.

25. Department of Health. *Community Mental Health Teams, Policy Implementation Guidance.* London: Department of Health; 2002.

26. Tyrer P, Morgan J, Van Horn E, *et al.* A randomised controlled study of close monitoring of vulnerable psychiatric patients. *Lancet* 1995; **345**(8952): 756–759.

27. Tyrer P, Evans K, Gandhi N, *et al.* Randomised controlled trial of two models of care for discharged psychiatric patients. *BMJ* 1998; **316**(7125): 106–109.

28. Thornicroft G, Wykes T, Holloway F, Johnson S and Szmukler G. From efficacy to effectiveness in community mental health services. PRiSM Psychosis Study 10. *Br. J. Psychiatry* 1998; **173**: 423–427.

29. Simmonds S, Coid J, Joseph P, Marriott S and Tyrer P. Community mental health team management in severe mental illness: a systematic review. *Br. J. Psychiatry* 2001; **178**: 497–502.

30. Tyrer S, Coid J, Simmonds S, Joseph P and Marriott S. *Community Mental Health Teams (CMHTs) for People With Severe Mental Illnesses and Disordered Personality (Cochrane Review)*. Oxford: Update Software; 2003.

31. Burns T. Generic versus specialist mental health teams. In Thornicroft G and Szmukler G (Eds.). *Textbook of Community Psychiatry*. Oxford: Oxford University Press; 2001: 231–241.

32. Sytema S, Micciolo R and Tansella M. Continuity of care for patients with schizophrenia and related disorders: a comparative south-Verona and Groningen case-register study. *Psychol. Med.* 1997; **27**(6): 1355–1362.

33. Holloway F and Carson J. Case management: an update. *Int. J. Soc. Psychiatry* 2001; **47**(3): 21–31.

34. Thornicroft G. The concept of case management for long-term mental illness. *Int. Rev. Psychiatry* 1991; **3**: 125–132.

35. Ziguras SJ and Stuart GW. A meta-analysis of the effectiveness of mental health case management over 20 years. *Psychiatr. Serv.* 2000; **51**(11): 1410–1421.

36. Ziguras SJ, Stuart GW and Jackson AC. Assessing the evidence on case management. *Br. J. Psychiatry* 2002; **181**: 17–21.

37. Mueser KT, Bond GR, Drake RE and Resnick SG. Models of community care for severe mental illness: a review of research on case management. *Schizophr. Bull.* 1998; **24**(1): 37–74.

38. Saarento O, Hansson L, Sandlund M, *et al.* The Nordic comparative study on sectorized psychiatry. Utilization of psychiatric hospital care related to amount and allocation of resources to psychiatric services. *Soc. Psychiatry Psychiatr. Epidemiol.* 1996; **31**(6): 327–335.

39. Hansson L, Muus S, Vinding HR, *et al.* The Nordic Comparative Study on Sectorized Psychiatry: contact rates and use of services for patients with a functional psychosis. *Acta Psychiatr. Scand.* 1998; **97**(5): 315–320.

40. Johnson S, Nolan F, Pilling S, *et al.* Randomised controlled trial of acute mental health care by a crisis resolution team: the north Islington crisis study. *BMJ* 2005; **331**(7517): 599.

41. Johnson S, Nolan F, Hoult J, *et al.* Outcomes of crises before and after introduction of a crisis resolution team. *Br. J. Psychiatry* 2005; **187**: 68–75.

42. Szmukler G and Holloway F. In-patient treatment. In Thornicroft G and Szmukler G (Eds.). *Textbook of Community Psychiatry*. Oxford: Oxford University Press; 2001: 321–337.

43. Johnstone P and Zolese G. Systematic review of the effectiveness of planned short hospital stays for mental health care. *BMJ* 1999; **318**(7195): 1387–1390.

44. Knapp M, Chisholm D, Astin J, Lelliott P and Audini B. The cost consequences of changing the hospital-community balance: the mental health residential care study. *Psychol. Med.* 1997; **27**(3): 681–692.

45. Quirk A and Lelliott P. What do we know about life on acute psychiatric wards in the UK? A review of the research evidence. *Soc. Sci. Med.* 2001; **53**(12): 1565–1574.

46. Tomov T. Central and Eastern European Countries. In Thornicroft G and Tansella M (Eds.). *The Mental Health Matrix. A Manual to Improve Services.* Cambridge: Cambridge University Press; 2001: 216–227.

47. Tansella M. Community psychiatry without mental hospitals – the Italian experience: a review. *J. R. Soc. Med.* 1986; **79**(11): 664–669.

48. Thornicroft G and Bebbington P. Deinstitutionalisation – from hospital closure to service development. *Br. J. Psychiatry* 1989; **155**: 739–753.

49. Shepherd G and Murray A. Residential care. In Thornicroft G and Szmukler G (Eds.). *Textbook of Community Psychiatry.* Oxford: Oxford University Press; 2001: 309–320.

50. Leff J. *Care in the Community. Illusion or Reality?* London: John Wiley & Sons, Ltd.; 1997.

51. Holloway F, Wykes T, Petch E and Lewis-Cole K. The new long stay in an inner city service: a tale of two cohorts. *Int. J. Soc. Psychiatry* 1999; **45**(2): 93–103.

52. van Wijngaarden GK, Schene A, Koeter M, *et al.* People with schizophrenia in five European countries: conceptual similarities and intercultural differences in family caregiving. *Schizophr. Bull.* 2003; **29**(3): 573–586.

53. Warner R. *Recovery from Schizophrenia,* 2nd edn. London: Routledge; 1994.

54. Warr P. *Work, Unemployment and Mental Health.* Oxford: Oxford University Press; 1987.

55. Social Exclusion Unit. *Mental Health and Social Exclusion.* London: Office of the Deputy Prime Minister; 2004.

56. Shepherd G. *Theory and Practice of Psychiatric Rehabilitation.* Chichester: John Wiley & Sons, Ltd; 1990.

57. Rosen A and Barfoot K. Day care and occupation: structured rehabilitation and recovery programmes and work. In Thornicroft G and Szmukler G (Eds.). *Textbook of Community Psychiatry.* Oxford: Oxford University Press; 2001: 296–308.

58. Catty J, Burns T and Comas A. *Day Centres for Severe Mental Illness (Cochrane Review).* The Cochrane Library, Issue 1. Oxford: Update Software; 2003.

59. Marshall M, Crowther R, Almaraz-Serrano A *et al.* Systematic reviews of the effectiveness of day care for people with severe mental disorders: (1) acute day hospital versus admission; (2) vocational rehabilitation; (3) day hospital versus outpatient care. *Health Technol. Assess.* 2001; **5**(21): 1–75.

60. Deci PA, Santos AB, Hiott DW, Schoenwald S and Dias JK. Dissemination of assertive community treatment programs. *Psychiatr. Serv.* 1995; **46**(7): 676–678.

61. Teague GB, Bond GR and Drake RE. Program fidelity in assertive community treatment: development and use of a measure. *Am. J. Orthopsychiatry* 1998; **68**(2): 216–232.

62. Scott J and Lehman A. Case management and assertive community treatment. In Thornicroft G and Szmukler G (Eds.). *Textbook of Community Psychiatry.* Oxford: Oxford University Press; 2001: 253–264.

63. Killaspy H, Bebbington P, Blizard R, *et al.* The REACT study: randomised evaluation of assertive community treatment in north London. *BMJ* 2006; **332**(7545): 815–820.

64. Marshall M and Lockwood A. Assertive community treatment for people with severe mental disorders (Cochrane Review). *The Cochrane Library, Issue 1.* Oxford: Update Software; 2003.

65. Phillips SD, Burns BJ, Edgar ER, *et al.* Moving assertive community treatment into standard practice. *Psychiatr. Serv.* 2001; **52**(6): 771–779.
66. Latimer EA. Economic impacts of assertive community treatment: a review of the literature. *Can. J. Psychiatry* 1999; **44**(5): 443–454.
67. Fiander M, Burns T, McHugo GJ and Drake RE. Assertive community treatment across the Atlantic: comparison of model fidelity in the UK and USA. *Br. J. Psychiatry* 2003; **182**: 248–254.
68. Burns T, Creed F, Fahy T, *et al.* Intensive versus standard case management for severe psychotic illness: a randomised trial. UK 700 Group. *Lancet* 1999; **353**(9171): 2185–2189.
69. Burns T, Fioritti A, Holloway F, Malm U and Rossler W. Case management and assertive community treatment in Europe. *Psychiatr. Serv.* 2001; **52**(5): 631–636.
70. Addington J, Coldham EL, Jones B, Ko T and Addington D. The first episode of psychosis: the experience of relatives. *Acta Psychiatr. Scand.* 2003; **108**(4): 285–289.
71. Raune D, Kuipers E and Bebbington PE. Expressed emotion at first-episode psychosis: investigating a carer appraisal model. *Br. J. Psychiatry* 2004; **184**: 321–326.
72. Kuipers E, Holloway F, Rabe-Hesketh S and Tennakoon L. An RCT of early intervention in psychosis: Croydon Outreach and Assertive Support Team (COAST). *Soc. Psychiatry Psychiatr. Epidemiol.* 2004; **39**(5): 358–363.
73. Petersen L, Jeppesen P, Thorup A, *et al.* A randomised multicentre trial of integrated versus standard treatment for patients with a first episode of psychotic illness. *BMJ* 2005; **331**(7517): 602.
74. Marshall M and Lockwood A. Early Intervention for psychosis. *Cochrane Database Syst. Rev.* 2004;(2): CD004718.
75. McGorry PD, Yung AR, Phillips LJ, *et al.* Randomized controlled trial of interventions designed to reduce the risk of progression to first-episode psychosis in a clinical sample with subthreshold symptoms. *Arch. Gen. Psychiatry* 2002; **59**(10): 921–928.
76. McGorry PD and Killackey EJ. Early intervention in psychosis: a new evidence-based paradigm. *Epidemiol. Psichiatr. Soc.* 2002; **11**(4): 237–247.
77. Friis S, Larsen TK, Melle I, *et al.* Methodological pitfalls in early detection studies – the NAPE Lecture 2002. Nordic Association for Psychiatric Epidemiology. *Acta Psychiatr. Scand.* 2003; **107**(1): 3–9.
78. Harrigan SM, McGorry PD and Krstev H. Does treatment delay in first-episode psychosis really matter? *Psychol. Med.* 2003; **33**(1): 97–110.
79. Larsen TK, Friis S, Haahr U, *et al.* Early detection and intervention in first-episode schizophrenia: a critical review. *Acta Psychiatr. Scand.* 2001; **103**(5): 323–334.
80. Warner R and McGorry PD. Early intervention in schizophrenia: points of agreement. *Epidemiol. Psichiatr. Soc.* 2002; **11**(4): 256–257.
81. Wiersma D, Kluiter H, Nienhuis FJ, Ruphan M and Giel R. Costs and benefits of hospital and day treatment with community care of affective and schizophrenic disorders. *Br. J. Psychiatry Suppl.* 1995;(27): 52–59.
82. Sledge WH, Tebes J, Wolff N and Helminiak TW. Day hospital/crisis respite care versus inpatient care, Part II: Service utilization and costs. *Am. J. Psychiatry* 1996; **153**(8): 1074–1083.

83. Sledge WH, Tebes J, Rakfeldt J, *et al.* Day hospital/crisis respite care versus inpatient care, Part I: Clinical outcomes. *Am. J. Psychiatry* 1996; **153**(8): 1065–1073.

84. Davies S, Presilla B, Strathdee G and Thornicroft G. Community beds: the future for mental health care? *Soc. Psychiatry Psychiatr. Epidemiol.* 1994; **29**(6): 241–243.

85. Sledge WH, Tebes J, Wolff N and Helminiak TW. Day hospital/crisis respite care versus inpatient care, Part II: Service utilization and costs. *Am. J. Psychiatry* 1996; **153**(8): 1074–1083.

86. Mosher LR. Soteria and other alternatives to acute psychiatric hospitalization: a personal and professional review. [Review] [48 refs]. *J. Nerv. Mental Disease* 1999; **187**(3): 142–149.

87. Killaspy H, Dalton J, McNicholas S and Johnson S. Drayton Park, an alternative to hospital admission for women in acute mental health crisis. *Psychiatr. Bull.* 2000; **24**: 101–104.

88. Catty J, Burns T, Knapp M, *et al.* Home treatment for mental health problems: a systematic review. *Psychol. Med.* 2002; **32**(3): 383–401.

89. Joy C, Adams C and Rice K. *Crisis Intervention for People With Severe Mental Illness (The Cochrane Library)*. Oxford: Update Software; 1998.

90. Glover G, Arts G and Babu KS. Crisis resolution/home treatment teams and psychiatric admission rates in England. *Br. J. Psychiatry* 2006; **189**(5): 441–445.

91. Sutherby K, Szmukler GI, Halpern A, *et al.* A study of 'crisis cards' in a community psychiatric service. *Acta Psychiatr. Scand.* 1999; **100**(1): 56–61.

92. Sutherby K and Szmukler GI. Crisis cards and self-help crisis initiatives. *Psychiatr. Bull.* 1998;(22): 4–7.

93. Sutherby K, Szmukler GI, Halpern A, *et al.* A study of 'crisis cards' in a community psychiatric service. *Acta Psychiatr. Scand.* 1999; **100**(1): 56–61.

94. Henderson C, Flood C, Leese M, *et al.* Effect of joint crisis plans on use of compulsory treatment in psychiatry: single blind randomised controlled trial. *BMJ* 2004; **329**(7458): 136.

95. Flood C, Byford S, Henderson C, *et al.* Joint crisis plans for people with psychosis: economic evaluation of a randomised controlled trial. *BMJ* 2006; **333**(7571): 729.

96. Shepherd G, Muijen M, Dean R and Cooney M. Residential care in hospital and in the community – quality of care and quality of life. *Br. J. Psychiatry* 1996; **168**(4): 448–456.

97. Trieman N, Smith HE, Kendal R and Leff J. The TAPS Project 41: homes for life? Residential stability five years after hospital discharge. Team for the Assessment of Psychiatric Services. *Community Ment. Health. J.* 1998; **34**(4): 407–417.

98. Chilvers R, Macdonald G and Hayes A. *Supported Housing for People With Severe Mental Disorders (Cochrane Review)*. Oxford: Update Software; 2003.

99. Nordentoft M, Knudsen HC and Schulsinger F. Housing conditions and residential needs of psychiatric patients in Copenhagen. *Acta Psychiatr. Scand.* 1992; **85**(5): 385–389.

100. Hafner H. Do we still need beds for psychiatric patients? An analysis of changing patterns of mental health care. *Acta Psychiatr. Scand.* 1987; **75**(2): 113–126.

101. Polak P and Warner R. The economic life of seriously mentally ill people in the community. *Psychiatr. Serv.* 1996; **47**(3): 270–274.

102. Lehman AF, Carpenter WT, Jr., Goldman HH and Steinwachs DM. Treatment outcomes in schizophrenia: implications for practice, policy, and research. *Schizophr. Bull.* 1995; **21**(4): 669–675.

103. Wiersma D, Nienhuis FJ, Slooff CJ, Giel R and De Jong A. Assessment of needs for care among patients with schizophrenic disorders 15 and 17 years after first onset of psychosis. *Epidemiol. Psichiatr. Soc.* 1997; **6**(1 Suppl): 21–28.

104. Latimer EA, Lecomte T, Becker DR, *et al.* Generalisability of the individual placement and support model of supported employment: results of a Canadian randomised controlled trial. *Br. J. Psychiatry* 2006; **189**: 65–73.

105. Cook JA, Leff HS, Blyler CR, *et al.* Results of a multisite randomized trial of supported employment interventions for individuals with severe mental illness. *Arch. Gen. Psychiatry* 2005; **62**(5): 505–512.

106. Thornicroft G, Rose D, Huxley P, Dale G and Wykes T. What are the research priorities of mental health service users? *J. Mental Health* 2002; **11**: 1–5.

107. Becker DR, Drake RE, Farabaugh A and Bond GR. Job preferences of clients with severe psychiatric disorders participating in supported employment programs. *Psychiatr. Serv.* 1996; **47**(11): 1223–1226.

108. Chamberlin J. User/consumer involvement in mental health service delivery. *Epidemiol. Psichiatr. Soc.* 2005; **14**(1): 10–14.

109. Drake RE, McHugo GJ, Bebout RR, *et al.* A randomized clinical trial of supported employment for inner-city patients with severe mental disorders. *Arch. Gen. Psychiatry* 1999; **56**(7): 627–633.

110. Priebe S, Warner R, Hubschmid T and Eckle I. Employment, attitudes toward work, and quality of life among people with schizophrenia in three countries. *Schizophr. Bull.* 1998; **24**(3): 469–477.

111. Lehman AF, Goldberg R, Dixon LB, *et al.* Improving employment outcomes for persons with severe mental illnesses. *Arch. Gen. Psychiatry* 2002; **59**(2): 165–172.

112. Burns T, Catty J, Becker T, *et al.* The effectiveness of supported employment for people with severe mental illness: a randomised controlled trial. *Lancet* 2007; **370** (9593): 1146–1152.

113. Thornicroft G and Tansella M. Balancing community-based and hospital-based mental health care. *World Psychiatry* 2002; **1**: 84–90.

114. Patel V and Sumathipala A. International representation in psychiatric literature: survey of six leading journals. *Br. J. Psychiatry* 2001; **178**: 406–409.

115. Isaakidis P, Swingler GH, Pienaar E, Volmink J and Ioannidis JP. Relation between burden of disease and randomised evidence in sub-Saharan Africa: survey of research. *BMJ* 2002; **324**(7339): 702.

6

The experience base for mental health care

Ann Law, Graham Thornicroft, and Michele Tansella

Distilling experience

In this chapter we shall present key issues which arise from everyday practice, so that these can be helpful to you as you try to implement better mental health care. In the previous chapters we have outlined contributions from the ethical base and from the evidence base. Here we discuss the third leg of this triangle: the experience base.

Our starting point for this chapter is our own accumulated experience from developing community-orientated mental health services in England and Italy over the last 20–30 years. We have organised what we have learned in relation to a series of key issues and challenges, as described below. We then contacted colleagues from across the world, asking them about their experiences in relation to these issues, using a simple, semi-structured questionnaire. We present here the replies from colleagues in 25 countries worldwide (from across Africa, the Americas, Asia, Australasia and Europe). The responses summarised in this chapter are from people who have very extensive national and international experience in implementing changes in mental health care, and whose details are given in the acknowledgements section. They were asked for their views on the proposals we made, on the basis of our own experience, whether they agreed or disagreed and to comment on how far their experiences corresponded with our own. These contributions, which have largely confirmed and validated our own initial views, are summarised in the following sections of this chapter, and are also used as examples to illustrate key points in other chapters. We are most grateful to them all. The points summarised in this chapter are discussed in more detail in other parts of this book.

The selection of these commentators is not unbiased, nor are their views entirely impartial. What, in fact, we have done is what often happens in ordinary clinical or managerial practice when an opportunity occurs to improve mental-health care: we have gone to people whose judgement we trust to ask for advice. This chapter will therefore present an overview of what this collective experience-based exercise reveals in terms of pragmatic approaches to service improvement.

A framework from experience

From our own experience we have provisionally concluded that the following issues are central to the development of balanced mental health services:

- Services need to reflect the priorities of service users and carers.
- Evidence supports the need for both hospital and community services.
- Services need to be provided close to home.
- Some services need to be mobile rather than static.
- Interventions need to address both symptoms and disabilities.
- Treatment has to be specific to individual needs.

> *Clients' priorities have to be accepted independent of the 'mental health care' system which is often technically orientated. [Germany]*

There is very strong international support from our colleagues for these ideas as central pillars to support service development. Many stressed the importance of the first point in particular, namely the need to ensure that services reflect the priorities of service-users and carers. Similarly, many experts agreed that there is a continuing, often limited role, for acute psychiatric beds, usually in general hospital settings, even when community services and teams have been fully developed.

> *In our experience, Turkey is at the very beginning period of implementing community care. As a result of the lack of community services, inpatient facilities are overloaded, cooperation with the patient is low.*

Those in low and middle income countries often described situations where none of these conditions currently apply. For example, if service-user/patient groups do not exist, then they are not available to be consulted or involved in planning. There was a strong consensus that in this vision there is no place for long-stay psychiatric hospitals in modern and balanced care.

> *Sarawak General Hospital where I worked before only has out-patient service, therefore community service is ultimately important as adjunct to the current service available. Mental institution carries strong stigma among the local and thus community service that being set up in a general hospital has done a great help to some of the patients that needed in-patient care. [Malaysia]*

General adult mental health care

Within the wider context of these broad guidelines, we shall discuss next the main categories of service which are necessary for comprehensive care. In Chapter 5 we described five key categories of service, all of which are necessary to provide a comprehensive range of local services:

- Out-patient/ambulatory clinics
- Community mental health teams
- Acute in-patient care
- Long-term residential care in the community
- Rehabilitation, work and occupation.

Across all countries there is very strong agreement that all these categories of care are necessary. In addition, it may be important to develop variations, or even separate forms of support, which are directly service-user-led, such as peer support workers, peer advocacy workers or self-help groups.

> The mental health care should however be complemented by peer support groups and other user-led activities. [Finland]

Pragmatically this means that for a service in transition, it is not necessary to delay reducing the size of a long-stay psychiatric hospital until all these components exist in the community. That would often be impossible because the main or the only source of funds for community services is from savings made at the large hospital as it reduces in size.

> However in developing countries it may not be possible to have 'community mental health teams'. The arguments often tend to go that if one doesn't have all the elements you mention, that people should be kept in long stay hospitals. [South Africa]

In fact, there is often a dilemma about whether to spend money on increasing the quality of care within large and usually neglected psychiatric hospitals, or rather on developing services outside hospital. In our experience the answer to this dilemma will need to be resolved according to local circumstances, but, in general, it is important to progressively move an increasing proportion of the whole mental health budget, and in many cases eventually the majority of the budget, to community-based services, while simultaneously bringing the quality of care in the (shrinking) institutions to an acceptable level. Here again there is a balance: too rapid a shift of resources can produce unstable and confused new clinical services that are unable to offer integrated care, especially to people with long-term mental disorders: too slow a process may not allow any momentum for change to be created.

> *Young psychiatrists explained to me that the place of a psychiatrist is in the hospital and the community is for the failed, incompetent ones! [Romania]*

Investment during the transition from a more hospital- to a more community-oriented system often needs a focus upon training to achieve individually orientated staff attitudes and practices (invisible inputs), for staff in hospital and community settings, rather than upon investment in the physical environment. The advantage of this way of setting priorities is that staff in the future, wherever they work, will have a more therapeutic and client-centred approach.

> *Many in-patient institutions do not provide any psychosocial rehabilitation, work and occupation to their patients and are rather 'warehouse hospitals' where patients are simply locked in wards with terrible conditions. In 2005 we started a project on involving patients to psychosocial rehabilitation and occupation and, according to numerous interviews with the staff and the patients, this had a very positive impact on participants' well-being.*

Stakeholders

In our view mental health services are best planned by bringing together the whole range of stakeholders who have an active interest in improving mental health care, including:

- Service-users
- Family members/carers
- Professionals (mental health and primary care)
- Other service provider groups, e.g. non-governmental organisations
- Policy makers
- Advocacy groups
- Planners.

There was very strong support for this view from colleagues across all countries, but there is also often frustration when this does not happen in practice.

> *But making it happen is still a dream in our country. These issues have been extensively discussed through local, state and federal assemblies called Mental Health Conferences. However, implementing policies is the next step. [Brazil]*

There is also a need to ensure that groups which are not powerful advocates for their own interests are also given equitable consideration in planning services.

> It is important to ensure equity and access to mental health services for all. Needs of 'invisible groups', such as illegal immigrants, victims of trafficking, prisoners, ethnic minorities (e.g. Roma people), can be forgotten, if not actively defended by any stakeholder. To ensure equity, politicians and public health officers should be involved in the planning. [Finland]

Indeed the involvement of stakeholders may be required under some circumstances by law.

> However, care must be taken to ensure that service-users are afforded more than a token place in these processes, and must be empowered and facilitated to do so. Under international law, such as the UN Standard Rules on the Equalization of Opportunities for Persons with Disabilities, people with disabilities have a right to participate in all decision-making that affects them. [Ireland]

At the same time it is clear that there is an 'asymmetry of information, lobby and power' [Germany] between professionals and service-users. Less powerful groups may need to take special measures to increase their influence. 'At least in Romania in order to survive NGOs have to be very aggressive to catch the eye of the media.' At the same time some particular stakeholders have the most powerful roles to either facilitate or veto service changes.

> My experience is that very important and powerful stakeholders in improving process are finance organisation[s] (Sickness insurance fund) and existing service providers (director of mental hospitals etc.). Time is necessary [to] change hospital directors and ... [this will be] very effective for reform. [Latvia]

What can be done where some key stakeholder groups do not exist? In this case it may be necessary to take a long-term view and for those controlling mental health financial resources to initiate and to support the growth of, for example, service-user and family member groups.

> In some countries though consumers and family members have been so disempowered and stigmatised that getting their meaningful participation is extremely difficult. Building up consumer groups who can talk on behalf of themselves and other consumers can be an extremely slow process. This can then lead to lack of any movement on service development while one 'waits for consumers to participate'. [South Africa]

Ten key challenges

From our experience in developing and working in community mental health services we have identified 10 key challenges facing people committed to improving mental health care, which are presented here in italics in the first box in each of the following 10 sections, followed by selected remarks upon each point from our 27 commentators from 25 countries.

Challenge 1. Anxiety and uncertainty

> *Creating new services necessarily produces uncertainty about the future. It is usually helpful if clear undertakings can be given, for example, guarantees to staff to avoid redundancies. It is an advantage to have some staff who prefer to work in hospital as such services will continue to be needed in future. Service leaders can help staff by openly supporting shared risk taking, and by allowing mistakes, as long as there is a learning/adaptation process at the same time.*

We have found very strong international agreement for these propositions. The challenge is to implement changes on the right tempo: *'Too fast will increase the anxiety for some persons, too slow will demotivate other people' [Belgium].* But risk taking may not be a strong feature of stable, often state sector, systems: *'most mental health professionals are employed in the public health services. The notion of risk taking does not fit with our daily experience' [Brazil].* One way to manage this need to motivate staff is to encourage a learning culture: *'Staff have to experience how care can be different … we think that one crucial element is a constructive work atmosphere where mistakes are transformed into better mental health care' [Germany].* A further way to deal with anxiety is to insist on manageable timetables for service changes. *'Schedules should be realistic and respected' [Greece].*

In addition, staff will usually find change more acceptable if it is broken down into smaller and more manageable steps: *'Anxiety about uncertainty of the outcome of a new service was inevitable, but we decided to take a small step at a time, and that really helped' [Malaysia].* A common mistake for senior managers and clinical staff is to tell junior staff *what* will change (in a new service structure), but not *why* the changes are taking place: *'It is helpful to clarify what changes will be undertaken and what that means for the staff' [Moldova].* In our experience most staff in mental health services do genuinely wish to contribute to better treatment and care, and for this reason it is vital to explain to all staff, sometimes in great detail, the *rationale* for service changes, before talking about more practical details: *'When we were planning new services the staff of the clinics had often been concerned about the changes and many, many questions were asked from them. It was obvious that responding to these concerns was very much helpful to all parties' [Tajikistan].*

Although guarantees of no redundancies, if possible, can be very helpful, for example through constructive discussions with trade unions, in low-resource countries there may be high staff vacancy rates and the question of redundancy does not arise: *'The system is so understaffed that any development would mean hiring new nurses, psychologists and social workers (at the moment we have almost none!)' [Romania]; 'Our main challenge is retaining staff in the context of critical staff shortages' [South Africa].*

> *The Board accepts that staff, users and carers will all make decisions which are risky in that they may not have predictable or definitely successful outcomes. Taking these, often difficult, decisions is a part of everyday practice. The Board fully supports staff in taking these decisions provided they are made responsibly by reference to the principles of good professional practice.*

> Examples of ensuring responsible risk taking include:
> - *Making use of the Care Programme Approach (case management and care planning) policy; crisis and contingency planning can help in arriving at a high risk decision and ensuring good communication*
> - *Risky decisions are discussed fully with key members of the team*
> - *Testing decisions with colleagues*
> - *Seeking advice from professional bodies*
> - *Seeking advice from Trust lawyers*
> - *Clear entries in the health care record should outline how the decision was made and the alternatives considered*
> - *Good note-keeping enables one to justify decisions.*
>   (Extract from South London and Maudsley NHS Foundation Trust Policy on Responsible Risk Taking)

Challenge 2. Lack of structure in community services

> *The change of service structure, and in particular developing more and smaller services away from the main hospital site, can run the risk of destroying established routines and structures. One of the positive functions of these routines is to reduce anxiety, and recognising this it may be important to develop, especially for a transitional period, even more structure and routine than is strictly necessary. This may include, for example, staff support groups, regular information-sharing meetings between managers and staff, and clear timetable of regular clinical meetings, as well as written operational policies and referral procedures.*

There is almost complete agreement on these points from all our colleagues. For example service-user-orientated procedures can offer postive structure in community care settings: *'In our experience, treatment and care plans are an excellent way to overcome anxiety (for patients, as well as carers and staff)'* *[Slovenia]; 'Structure and routine is helpful in times of change, as long as this does not lead to more management and documentation' [Germany]; 'Written operational policies are referral procedures have proved themselves to be very helpful' [Tajikistan].*

On the other hand, one site expressed a slightly different emphasis, and particularly stressed the need to avoid re-establishing old structures and routines in new settings: *'The abandonment of routines does not have to re-create immediately new routines. The key issue is to overcome the institutional thinking and to open a process of participation and communication, with power shifts and democracy ... written procedures, in a period of change, are unuseful because they are formulated a priori with no connections with the new emerging from change' [Italy].* Yet most experts do take the view that *new* structures and routines are necessary, especially in periods of transition: *'Developing new routines and structures must be performed during the period when a certain uncertainty and chaos must be dealt with. New routines and organisation do not just pop up fixed and ready to use' [Sweden].*

Challenge 3. How to initiate new developments?

Often the biggest challenge facing stakeholders in beginning a process of reform is that it is difficult to imagine how the mental health system could possibly be different. An invaluable way to begin is by visiting other places which have begun or completed the development of community-based care. It is often helpful to borrow a copy of some of their basic tools, such as timetables, assessment forms, job descriptions or operational policies. As a local service development plan develops, it is often important to allocate each task to a person or group and to set a deadline for its completion, along with a mechanism, such as the next meeting of the planning group, to see whether tasks have been completed or not. It may need to become clear to staff that it does matter, for example to their salary or to their promotion, whether they fulfil the agreed tasks or not.

Among the many responses that supported these views were those that stressed the need to see new services elsewhere at first hand: *'Visiting other places where mental health care has been changed is more important than hearing speeches and reading reports' [Germany].* Who should go? This depends on the purpose of the visit. For national/regional policy change then senior policy-makers, finance officers and officials will be the key personnel. For local level changes, such as developing community mental health teams, then a full range of practitioners will need to be involved: *'Taking a full team to visit and allowing people to interact with their counterparts at different levels may prove more beneficial than just taking the leaders' [South Africa].*

Which services should be visited? In our view it is especially important to visit examples of evidence-based models of care: *'There is a lot of money spent in Europe to visit different models, practices, many times bad and worse practices ... Evidence-based projects should be implemented instead of so many local models with low effectiveness' [Hungary].* Taking every opportunity of taking concrete examples home from visits, such as operational policies, is often found to be very helpful: *'Bringing home copies of their tools and protocols was tremendously helpful and saved a lot of time. Adjusting them to the local settings was an important part too' [Tajikistan].* Even so, on reflection some of these documents may turn out not to be suitable for local adaptation, but can stimulate discussion on what is required locally: *'They brought many basic tools with them, but none was really used later. However, their personal experience and training has yielded progress in terms of organisation, flexibility and coordination of tasks' [Slovenia].*

Care is needed in choosing where to visit, and staff from a low- or medium-resource country may plan to go to a fairly similar country and not a high-resources site: *'We have largely followed this way (visiting other experiences either in other parts of Greece or abroad) and it was very helpful indeed. However, there is [a] trap in this: if the mental health system we visit is much different from ours, then this creates disappointment to the visitors ("we'll never achieve such a level")' [Greece].*

After such visits, many countries have developed pilot projects, initially at one site, to test out if the new model of care can be successfully adapted to the local circumstances: *'In our country we first passed through a pilot phase, initiating new developments in the capital of Nicosia, with staff already experienced through their training to similar initiatives. Once successful, new developments were initiated in other Districts with staff exposed to Nicosia experience' [Cyprus].*

Putting such plans into action will usually mean developing, not just an overall policy, but also a very specific implementation plan: *'Having operational plans with deadlines and consequences if things are not done is critical' [South Africa].* At the same time important practical issues, such as staff salary levels, which may act as positive or negative incentives to change have to be tackled directly: *'What is also necessary is to ban differences, for example, in Romania there are huge salary differences according to the setting people work [in]. Those working in hospital earn 20–30% more and taking into account the bonus for night shifts even 50% which is dissuasive for those nurses who would like [to] come in[to] community teams!' [Romania].*

So the main reasons for visits to other services is twofold: to see ideas in practice and, from one's own direct experience, what it is possible to do, and to learn from specific aspects of practice elsewhere, and then to adapt this for local benefit: *'There is always something unique and a local flavour which cannot be copied'* [Sweden]; *'Every country should be adapting models for the local situation'* [Latvia]. In other words, *'all models are wrong, but some are useful!'* [1].

Challenge 4. How to manage opposition within the mental health system

Commonly there will be a range of staff views on proposals to change the care system. Many opportunities may be necessary to involve the range of staff, including a widespread process of consultation, with planning groups including diverse opinions. Linking local specific proposals to generally agreed plans, such as the World Health Organisation Declarations, can put your services in a wider context, and help to create a sense of the inevitability of change.

Again these views gained strong support across the range of experts consulted: *'It makes sense to stress the inevitability of change'* [Belgium]. Sometimes the key message may need to be explained repeatedly to importance target groups: *'It's a repetition principle. Everything must evolve: minds and actions'* [France]. As in Challenge 3, explaining the rationale for change may convince some staff to add their support to change: *'Linking proposals to human rights norms can also put services into a wider context'* [Ireland]. Quite often a senior member of staff, typically a senior official or a medical hospital director is initially unpersuaded by the arguments for change: *'Very important is to include this person in the reform process'* [Latvia].

If possible, identify changes which are to everyone's advantage: *'Try to identify and propose policies/changes that would make everybody better off (though that might be hard), or at least would be politically and economically feasible. When proposing a change identify the winners and the losers of the new policy and look what can be done for those who will be hurt by the policy. In my experience job security of the staff was one of the most important issues'* [Moldova].

Yet it is clear that some changes will need substantial changes in professional practice: *'In Romania the opposition might come from some psychiatrists, for whom a change could mean a menace for their income, status and power. Pressure from abroad is always helpful. For example to depenalise homosexuality it took almost ten years of pressure from the EU Parliament!!!'*

The value of external policy and practice recommendations from bodies such as the World Health Organisation is more controversial. In high-income countries these seem to be of less importance: *'I haven't found WHO declarations useful since the service models we develop are very context-dependent. What works in Glasgow, where the GP is an important part of the referral and treatment system, for example, will not be relevant in Philadelphia, where the GP is rarely part of the process'* [USA]. In a similar vein: *'I would place the primary evidence always on an evidence-based vision and testing things against that. Falling back on authorities such as WHO is useful but not powerful. [It] may induce yawning behaviour in some'* [New Zealand]. Nevertheless, all the low- and medium-resources countries give a high value to these international guidelines, especially if they are adapted to the local situation: *'Adhering to WHO declarations can help in managing opposition ... Seek the support of masses using media ... Under these conditions [it] would be hard for the opposition to vote against the change'* [Moldova].

Often, after lengthy discussion, a number of staff will make it clear that despite all the arguments for developing community services, they wish to remain working on in-patient units. In the balanced care model that we describe in this book there is a clear need for some (limited) acute in-patient facilities (usually in general hospitals) and in this case there is a continuing need for specialists in acute in-patient treatment and care. On some occasions significant numbers of staff may be reluctant to proceed to service change: *'At times where there is strong resistance one may need to move more slowly than one would wish and show "local" successes, but having the international agreements helps a lot'* [South Africa].

Ultimately, however, some staff may simply refuse to take part in service changes which are generally agreed: *'There will always be a minority of staff members who are not willing or able to give up the old routines, both in community and hospital settings. These persons should be given the advice to make a career change'* [Netherlands], or in some cases this may be an appropriate time for the retirement of such staff.

Challenge 5. Opposition from neighbours

> *Neighbours will often have reservations, or may protest against plans for new mental health facilities in their locality. There is a dilemma here between maintaining the confidentiality of patients, and so not telling neighbours in advance about the new residents, or trying to engage support of neighbours through information-sharing and consultation. Our view is that involving neighbours throughout the process of developing into services is usually the better long-term option.*

Interestingly, there is little international agreement on these issues. The experience of our international colleagues lies across the whole spectrum from completely informing neighbours to telling them nothing before a new residential facility opens in their local area.

In favour of involving local residents in some cases is the legal necessity to do so: *'New non-governmental organisation projects need to register with the local government, and communities then have an opportunity to comment on the favourability of such projects in their areas' [South Africa].* The status of a particular project may also have a positive effect: *'We have not gone to the stage of putting our patients into community living in neighbourhood as yet. We are now in the process of doing this and we admit we have some resistance from the neighbour but we manage to overcome it by informing them that this is [a] government project' [Malaysia].* Indeed not engaging neighbours can lead to greater difficulties later on: *'In many places in the Netherlands we have seen the detrimental effects of not engaging neighbours in planning new facilities.'* If there is advance discussion with neighbours, its nature needs to be made clear in an honest way: *'I think that at times so-called consultation is nothing other than courtesy or information giving. In other words one will go ahead regardless. One needs to be clear at the start whether one is merely informing the community or really consulting them. I was recently called to give evidence in a case where the community were told they were part of a consultation process but when they objected the plans proceeded anyway. The community were furious that they were lied to. In this case I think the whole "consultation" process did far more harm than good!' [South Africa].*

To some extent the quality of the new facility may affect the judgements of neighbours: *'Another thing [that is] important to my opinion is the quality of the facility: the better it is, the easier will become part of the local community' [Greece].* But such early warning approaches also have their dangers: *'At the beginning of the process we have tried to involve the neighbours actively from the beginning. Because of the existing stigma, a number of our efforts failed' [Cyprus]; 'The "not in my backyard phenomenon" should never be underestimated' [Sweden].*

For this reason, many colleagues feel strongly that it is unhelpful to inform neighbours about the nature of a new community mental health facility in advance: *'So in Greece we have adopted the "hit and run" approach: first the facility is established, and immediately after neighbours get informed.'* Indeed there is a sound theoretical reason for this approach, namely the social contact theory that an effective way to reduce stigma is to have direct personal contact with a person in the stigmatised group [2;3]: *'I can add from my personal experience that building inter-personal relations with service users is very helpful. I think direct contact with users who are very nice persons is the best way to reduce neighbours' fear about service users' [Kyrgyzstan].*

Indeed a decision not to give advance notice to neighbours can be seen as one aspect of mainstreaming people with mental illness and related disabilities: *'Patients in our group homes never disturbed their neighbours or at least not more than other citizens and we see no need to define them as "special" in*

advance. We find these gentle warnings to be an obstacle to their actual integra-
tion into the local community. Patients should have the same opportunities to be
included as everybody else. We have established group homes with no specific
preparation and when the neighbours actually met the residents, they found out
that they were perfectly compatible and generally accepted them in their environ-
ments. Each misunderstanding and all questions were immediately discussed
with the support staff. This is in line with the anti-stigma research findings,
namely that direct contact improves attitudes and diminishes fears more than
any type of education' [Slovenia].

Whatever the stage at which neighbours are informed, or become aware of
the nature of the new facility, it is very important to take seriously their views: *'It*
is not necessary to prepare the neighbours too much in [advance], but that it is
very important to listen very carefully to their experiences once the new mental
health facility is operative. Honour their very specific expertise. If they signal
problems, take them serious[ly] and keep them informed about the measures that
will be undertaken to solve the problems' [Belgium]; 'Neighbours have to expe-
rience that things are "under control"' [Germany]. In a few low-resource countries this issue is not currently important because community facilities have not
yet been developed: *'We have never been confronted with this problem. I do not*
think in urban areas it will be a problem!' [Romania].

In all cases the ultimate aim will be to foster good neighbourly relations
between people in the community care home and local residents: *'It will*
promote a patient-friendly environment in the neighbourhood and in many
cases neighbours will be willing to help to the mental health facilities, to bring
food to the patients on religious and other holidays' [Tajikistan].

Challenge 6. Financial obstacles

Although some policy-makers, politicians or managers may see a move from
hospital towards community care as a cost-saving process, the experience of
many countries is that money can only be saved by reducing the quality of
care. It is therefore essential to monitor very closely the resources available to
mental services, and to ensure that no monies mysteriously become lost in the
process! One very valuable asset that can be released in changing the system of
care is the value of land and buildings occupied by the large psychiatric
hospitals. It is important to establish whether you can retain the money
realised by their rental or sale to use for new staff and facilities. Wherever
possible keep maximum flexibility in your mental health service budgets, and
share these budgets with other agencies if this is an advantage to you.

Money is critical for mental health care. To start with first principles: the
purpose of balancing hospital and community care is *not* to reduce the mental

health budget. Rather it is to provide the best possible services with the resources available. Indeed, as we shall discuss in more detail in Chapter 10 (regarding financial inputs), mental illnesses contribute 12% of the global burden of disease, yet worldwide only 2% of all health care expenditure is dedicated to mental health care. In this case it is clear that the overall proportion of the health budget spent on services for people with mental illnesses is, in most countries, grossly inadequate.

In relation to moving long-stay patients from large psychiatric institutions to community facilities, the evidence from evaluations carried out in high-resource countries shows that where this is done reasonably well, overall it is cost-neutral [4;5]. Indeed there is no evidence that comprehensive mental health care costs less than long-stay psychiatric hospitals. On the other hand, there is no support from research for the common idea that block treatment in hospital is more cost-effective (unless it is lower quality care): *'Some politicians believe that big hospitals might be more cost efficient benefiting from the economy of scale (having a single laboratory, using more efficiently the medical equipment (MRIs, CT scans, etc.), having greater negotiation power with pharmaceutical companies and contractors, using more efficiently the staff' [Moldova]*. The main point is that reshaping a service should not be seen as a cost-saving exercise: *'It is essential that creating a community mental health service is not a cost saving issue. The evidence suggests that institution-based mental health care is as expensive as a community mental health service system. The main point is flexibility in your mental health service budget' [Germany]*.

At the same time, such service changes can be used as the occasions to make budget cuts: *'However, even though money has been saved through the reduction of chronic hospital beds, there has not been a commensurate increase in community mental health services. Our community mental health clinics see more and more patients with fewer staff, and the development of NGO services has been slow. This is the very situation that mental health professionals warned would happen, and our health department has stopped further bed reductions for the moment' [South Africa]*.

One important financial issue is whether the total resources available for mental health care, for example for a local area, can be identified and protected (sometimes called 'ring-fenced'): *'I think a critical issue in our situation is the fact that we do not have a "ring-fenced" mental health care budget. The only identifiable budgets are those for psychiatric hospitals and chronic care institutions provided by a private company … part of the reason for using non-governmental organisations was that this was a way to ring-fence the money' [South Africa]*. This is a very important issue, because where such budgetary protection is not maintained then it is very common to see mental heath budgets lost to other medical departments: *'General hospital acute units have to compete for resources with other disciplines within each hospital, and usually lose out in the process' [South Africa]*.

The resale value of the land and buildings occupied by long-stay hospitals depends upon its location, condition and reputation, and often the value cannot be realised to use for other mental health services locally: *'Pretty often mental hospitals are in very bad condition and out of [the centre] of [the] city [the] value of land and building is very low' [Latvia].*

A very important, but rarely discussed, challenge in some countries is the inappropriate use of healthcare funds: *'Because of corruption, it is often the case that monies mysteriously become lost in the process! Whenever there is more money in the health service budgets there are some people who would like to appropriate this money.'* Another example makes a similar point: *'I was working in a large hospital where the chief was interested in keeping the hospital as the main source of care in the country, so he would have a large budget pocketing every year a part of the hospital money. He used to manipulate staff's opinion regarding mental health reforms telling them that the structural reforms would mean closure of many psychiatric wards and unemployment for most of them, consequently still now there is a resistance to structural changes of the mental health [care system].'*

A further key issue is whether local mental health resources are separated between, for example, health and social service budgets, or are integrated to allow greater flexibility in how they are invested in a range of local facilities and services: *'In Germany there is a pioneering project "Regionales Psychiatrie-Budget" (regional psychiatric budget) covering the mental health care of a whole region and enabling different providers to cooperate.'* One implication of this is that financial controls are agreed at the local level so that these funds can be used imaginatively to support agreed service changes. *'There are many different, creative ways of classifying aspects of the expenditure' [New Zealand].* But this is not always the case: *'Unfortunately, in Greece all financial aspects of the health matters are managed at [the] ministerial level. So, there should first become possible the decentralisation of resources management.'* Where this budgetary integration does occur it can produce very positive results: *'In Cyprus, budget for mental health services comes yearly from the government. Any decrease in the portion dedicated to in-patients results in the increase of the proportion for community services. There is still a need to supervise a good allocation of the money, though.'*

Challenge 7. System rigidity

> *One of the organisational features of large institutions is their hierarchical nature and the rigidity of their procedures. In community systems it is possible to adopt a more flexible approach to how staff are used. For example, secondments to other services, or periods of shadowing key members of staff can be useful to develop new skills and roles. Sometimes it is helpful to make joint appointments, where one post is shared between two organisations.*

There is common ground among virtually all commentators that one of the hallmarks of a community-based approach is the ability to adopt a more flexible approach to care than is usual in large institutions: '*I agree that large institutions are rigidity. Decentralization will help give more human, personal relationship between professionals and users and establish competition between stakeholders for better care*' *[Latvia].* Several colleagues particularly emphasised that such flexibilities should be used to keep patients at home as far as possible: '*Community systems are more flexible and could provide more community oriented care. In other words rather than taking [a] patient out of community and locking him/her up in a ward it is better to keep him/her in the community, with family and help not only with medical treatment but with finding a job, obtaining appropriate vocational training if needed, renting a room, making new friends, creating self supporting groups, etc. Community organizations also have more flexibility in making staff changes according to the needs of the patients: if they need more medical care – hire more psychiatrists, nurses, psychologists, if [they need] more help with social skills – hire more social workers, if [there are] problems with the law – contract more lawyers, etc.*' *[Moldova].* Some extended this to consider system flexibility in terms of the networking of service components: '*New ways of work, new attitudes, different patient-staff relationships, different risk-taking, and "networking" manager skills should be trained for staff*' *[Hungary].*

On the other hand, some were more sceptical: '*I find you very optimistic! Much depends upon managers' attitudes on how a service should run and at what level [it] should collaborate with other system components. Anyway, it's sure that [a] community mental health system needs to function in a different way than a large institution*' *[Greece].* Another pitfall is that of deterioration in community service: '*But community services are prone to becoming "institutionalized" in the sense of rigidity in their approach. Flexibility, human rights protection and personal involvement of staff are to be maintained through education, team work and regular supervision. We also think that the training of mental health staff is a crucial issue and that it needs to be reviewed and improved in keeping with evidence-based practice and mental health needs of the population*' *[Slovenia].* Further, it is the experience of many countries that they have not (yet) attempted to implement such changes: '*This is a very good idea, but we have not tried this yet*' *[Turkey]*; and '*[w]e have not been confronted with this situation! Your suggestion seems sensible*' *[Romania]*; '*Agree. However, there are no adequate community systems in Tajikistan yet to enable me to comment based on my own experience.*'

A basic question is whether there are resources on the ground which can be used at all, let alone flexibly: '*We have tried to do this with our community psychiatrists, [who] have been responsible for supervising acute psychiatric units in regional hospitals. This allows patients to be followed from community to hospital and back, and also gives the practitioners some variety in terms of their work, but is still not ideal due to the severe staff shortages in both regional hospitals and community mental health services' [South Africa].*

Challenge 8. Boundaries and barriers

As community mental health systems tend to be more complex than their hospital predecessors, it is vital that senior staff can maintain an overall view of the system as a whole. Individual components of service, for example clinical teams, must not be allowed to define their roles in isolation. They must be required to negotiate with other clinical teams to agree how they will put into practice a joint responsibility for all those patients who need to care. One way to manage inevitable ongoing boundary discussions about who does what is to have regular and frequent meetings between the leaders of all the clinical teams which serve a particular area.

Most commentators agreed with this core message, but with some variations of emphasis: *'It may be meaningful to even appoint one coordinator with respect to the content of care, [who] overlooks the totality of care and can more profoundly work out a long-term perspective. The development and permanent practice of a shared vision on care is very important in my opinion. Here again the role of leaders is crucial' [Belgium].* Indeed, the importance of clearly defined leadership was frequently mentioned: *'Agree, but I would also stress the need for overarching leadership built on commonly agreed local mental health strategy. Lack of such a leadership leads to lack of coordination, fragmentation of services, service gaps and doubling of efforts, and usually also to a dominance of specialised services over basic services and increased total costs' [Finland].*

On the other hand, although co-ordinated meetings were valued, these need not be too often!: *'But be careful to the time wasted in meetings... One of our concrete device: the phone conference between every unit, every morning, [lasts] half an hour' [France]; 'It is a common "disease" to engage in a "meeting culture" with many interesting issues being discussed, but many practical problems not being solved. In Germany, in recent years, quality management programmes in psychiatry are increasingly smiled at because they too often have nothing to do with clinical reality and serve administrative ends only.'* Such co-ordinating mechanisms are a part of a wider shift from one-to-one clinical contact to a model of multi-disciplinary team-working: *'Also sharing views, co-managing problems, and developing a sense of communality, can help to change, especially overcoming a concept of responsibility of individuals in favour of a responsibility of the team' [Italy].*

Even so, other contextual factors limit how far such flexibilities are possible in some countries: *'In post-soviet countries one of the main obstacle[s] and barrier[s] for changing is corruption in mental health system.'* Beyond individual or systematic corruptions, there may be structural arrangements that encourage competition and discourage co-operation and integration: *'The Slovene government has put mental health teams in the health, social and NGO sector in a competitive position, since they are all trying to obtain public funds and so their cooperation is not that strong. We believe that the mental health network should be carefully planned so as to avoid competition that impedes cooperation'* [Slovenia].

Indeed, in some countries there may be multiple, concurrent factors that tend to produce system fragmentation: *'There are a host of client-related challenges to take into account, e.g. disincentives to employment in the disability pension system, multiple points of entry into care that make coordinated community care difficult or impossible, lack of correspondence between the philosophy of the funders and the philosophy of the caregivers, lack of universal health insurance, lack of integration between hospital and community care, lack of academic involvement in provision of community services for the seriously ill, and distortion of psychiatric diagnostic practices by insurance/funding pressures'* [USA].

Challenge 9. Maintain morale

> *The morale of mental health staff is usually found to be low wherever the study takes place! In addition morale may be particularly difficult during times of system change. Managers may therefore need to make special arrangements, during these transitional periods, to boost morale, for example by paying attention to social events, by communicating successes and by taking any excuse to throw a party!*

Creating and maintaining high staff morale is universally recognised as vital to an effective mental health service, both the morale of individual staff members, and developing a strong reputation as a modern and professional team. All commentators agreed with this point: *'Staff burnout is an important challenge in the US'; 'Staff morale is essential. The higher the staff morale the easier it is to fill vacancies and to attract well trained professionals ... being perceived as a service meeting high professional standards (and providing specific interventions) and not as a team dealing with "disturbed persons" may provide the best protection against burn-out'* [Germany].

At the same time, there are cultural differences in what helps staff morale: *'Social events and parties don't fit with the local culture. Frequent exposure to success stories of other countries by exchange of visits may be more successful'* [Cyprus]; *'Managers' attitudes and beliefs are crucial, as they – willing or not – have the role of models for the rest of the staff. Much depends on them. If they are [keen on] system change, they can find many ways to boost staff's morale!'* [Greece]; *'One of the way[s] to increase the morale level is court cases. For example cases against slavery. In our country [for] many years patients were abused as slaves. We made efforts to appeal to the court. We couldn't get success in slave cases. However it was widely known to public through media. Finally we have success with court case against Kyrgyz Government.'* Gender-related issues may also be very important: *'In Slovenia, the largest portion of the personnel [is] women with children, and many have financial difficulties. That is why we are very enthusiastic in communicating success, but we do not invite them to parties very often.'*

The context for change is that in many countries, staff feel that mental healthcare has been historically neglected compared with other areas of medical practice: *'In Ireland, the mental health services are often described by the professionals operating within the system as the "Cinderella" of the health services, i.e. under-resourced and lacking political commitment, and one of the consequences of this is low morale. Mental health services are arguably more dependent on their human resources than other health sectors. Therefore, staff need to be made aware that their work is highly valued'; 'Maintaining morale of staff in psychiatry, be it in hospital or community setting is of great importance, because generally working in psychiatry is stigmatizing' [Malaysia].*

Several colleagues particularly highlighted the importance of clear and committed leadership to increase morale: *'There are crucial role of directors of facilities. Directors must clear[ly] explain all steps in [the] changing process ... that all staff is necessary for future work in new facilities and system' [Latvia]; 'I would suggest as well choosing leaders of the new organizations that are passionate about their work and who can inspire the staff' [Moldova]; 'To maintain the morale, it can also help to call in a consultant to manage the changing process and to channel (canalise) the resistance and low morale. It is also important to detect the persons that install or strengthen the negative morale, to listen to them, to validate their perspective but to try to give them a constructive role in the changing process' [Belgium].* One of the tasks of strong leadership is to clarify what is expected of staff: *'Morale gets better at the point when future tasks are defined. The worst burnout is caused by uncertainty about future system changes. The staff are connected and satisfied by our experience when they find their work important and fruitful. At least in our environment, this seems to be much more important than providing for good social communication' [Slovenia].*

Countries were less consistent on the question of whether social events for staff are helpful to support good staff morale: *'It is important to keep the morale of the staff up. I would suggest activities together i.e. once a week informal meetings at the end of the day or in the morning to have tea or donuts together would help to bring the morale up' [Moldova]; 'We used to make a lot of parties in the inpatient ward for non-psychotic patients which have been closed down [since] March 31, 2006. Had dinners outside, celebrated birthdays and farewells of rotating residents etc. The New Year parties were especially traditional and our staff had the highest morale in the hospital' [Turkey].* Yet it still needs to be clear that staff morale is a second goal which serves the primary purpose of better mental health for people with mental illness: '*I don't agree with Challenge 9, where you suggest staff social events are a good way to maintain staff morale. I believe that putting the client first and developing excellent services that the workers can be proud of is the best way to defeat burnout*' [USA].

A further way to enhance team morale is to visit other centres, for example abroad. This can have several advantages: to realise that one's own problems occur also elsewhere, to promote better social contact between staff team members, to learn directly from the practical experiences of others, and for the staff to be given some valuable reward for their commitment to the service, often over years or decades: '*For people in [a] developing country being able to attend a conference "overseas" and to use the opportunity to see successful projects elsewhere is an excellent motivator*' [South Africa].

Challenge 10. What is the right answer?

> *There is no right answer! Although there are a large number of mental health service models and theories, these are best seen as suggestions for what might help you in your particular situation. Maintain as much flexibility as you can in the new system, because you will make mistakes and need to change the service as it develops. The best guide about whether your mental health services are going in the right direction is the feedback you receive from service-users and family members about how far their preferences and needs are being responded to.*

It is common for those starting a process of mental health service change to believe that someone else, in some other place, knows exactly what should be done. In this book we try to describe general principles which will help you, but we also suggest that each local setting needs to find its own specific way to better mental health care: '*There may be no right answer, but there are some important principles which are fairly universal. For example, measuring performance against meeting needs; looking for ways to improve continuity of care; service commitment to random audit based quality assurance with Donabedian loops; service commitment to a recovery approach and attending to the consumer perspective*' [New Zealand].

The central importance of supporting, seeking and using feedback from service-users and family members was welcomed by almost all of our correspondents: '*I agree that the service users and their families are the most important criterion of evaluation (touchstone)*' [Belgium]; '*Feedback from service users and family members is extremely helpful. We think that you have to actively seek feedback in order not to have to rely upon reports of a highly selected user group.*

There is no easy and no single answer, and change processes have to take place in an ongoing and continuous manner' [Germany].

This perspective is based on an understanding that staff do not know all the answers: *'I agree under the condition that mental health services are ready to receive this feedback and have the mechanisms for that. This means that they have learned that they are not the "knowledge keepers"' [Greece].* Even so, such feedback may not be readily available: *'But there are times that services users and family members make no comments' [Cyprus].* A dilemma is that in social and health systems which have been relatively closed, staff and patients may not be able to imagine any other way to provide or receive care: *'Many families are for the moment at least partisan of seclusion as often as they are confronted with difficult situations. And there are even patients whose reproach toward professionals is that while manic or psychotic we did not put them in closed wards or who are not interested in discussing medication and for whom it is the psychiatrist's duty to decide' [Romania].* In fact we think that active dissent from service-users is a strong sign that higher standards are expected and needed: *'But I believe that even good services receive many complaints and I find expressed dissatisfaction to be a measure of quality. Patients often agree with every service offered because of their low expectations and low self esteem. Good services are those which empower them in a way that they are able to recognise our mistakes, which inevitably do happen' [Slovenia].*

Feedback can be based on comments or complaints received, or it can be formally invited, for example with service-user satisfaction surveys: *'Having some more formal evaluation – including feedback from users – also helps to confirm that one is going in the "right" direction, or points out areas where different approaches may be needed. People like to be part of a formal evaluation' [South Africa].* It is often the case that, before feedback can be received, statutory services need to invest time and money to support the creation and initial survival of service-user groups: *'Recently, a consumer advocacy group has been established in our province. It is our intention to engage with them to identify critical areas which need to improve, and to present a united front to lobby for the resources we need' [South Africa].* In this way, over time, advocacy groups can join forces with staff to lobby for more resources allocation to mental health care, and often politicians are more moved and persuaded by individuals who have personal experience of mental illness than by staff, whom they may suspect of being motivated for reasons of self-interest.

We therefore conclude that you need to have a sceptical view of what experts say and write!: *'There is no right or wrong answer. Your service development is based on your needs, your resources, your outcome and your continuing improvement ... Every model has to be flexible to the local culture and availability of human resource at the time' [Malaysia]; 'The "right answer" depends on what we would like to achieve. Traditional views, always present, can push changes toward too many compromises. Only a new, hopeful, strong vision of change can help that flexibility does not become a compromise. Even users and family members can't know what is the right answer (see many researches about good satisfaction with poor services: people don't know what can be done in a different way!)' [Italy].*

Lessons learned

What are the overall lessons that our group of colleagues, experts in developing community mental health services from 25 countries worldwide, can condense for others to learn from? Here we summarise what we consider to be the three most important overall issues that were reported by the expert group. First, there is a strong view that robust service changes, improvements that will last, *'take time' [Belgium].* Part of the reason for this is that staff will need to be persuaded that change is likely to bring improvements for patients, and indeed their scepticism is a positive asset, to act as a buffer against changes that are too rapid or too frequent. The next reason for not rushing change is that to succeed, services are likely to need the support of many organisations and agencies, which have to be identified and included gradually, at the start of each cycle of service changes. Those which are, or which feel, excluded are likely to oppose change, sometimes successfully. Further, in situations where health service changes may be a topic for political debate, it is usually necessary to build a cross-party consensus on the mental health strategy so that it will continue intact if the government changes. Again this will often take time to achieve.

Time is also needed to progress from the initiation stage of a change to the *consolidation phase.* Typically at the early stages of service reform a charismatic individual or small group will champion the main proposals, and recruit support from stakeholder groups and from others with influence within the health care system. In Eastern European countries, for example, the medical director/superintendents of the psychiatric hospital will, in practice, hold a veto for or against change: *'Our mistake was that we misunderstood the great role and authority of directors of mental hospitals.'* But after a series of initiatives, such as creating mental health day centres in the larger cities of a country, the mental health system needs to systematise these changes so that they can continue over many years. In this subsequent phase it is often true that charismatic leaders go on to new challenges, and the people who are most useful are those who are able to patiently consolidate the new organisation, and to establish consortia that are viable in the long term: *'Create a coalition of organisations and individuals that support the idea and bring together the resources of the members of the coalition (voters, money for mental health campaigns, personal connections with policy makers and the media)' [Moldova].* For example, these less visible individuals will set up proper supervision for staff, ensure the regular maintenance of buildings, arrange for personnel to undergo regular training, set up multi-agency working groups to identify and fix day-to-day problems in the running

Patterns of care (1979–2006)
South-Verona psychiatric case register
(Ratios × 1.000)

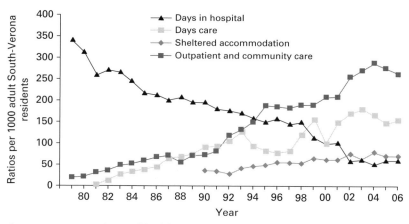

Figure 6.1 Patterns of mental health service provision in Verona, 1979–2006.

of the services, establish and take part in consultation or partnership meetings
with service-users/consumers and with family members, and monitor that the
services run properly within their allocated budgets: *'Leadership should not be
dependent too much on charisma of single individuals but on real accountability
to a larger group of people, and definitely to the wider community' [Italy].* An
example of the timescale required is the pattern of service changes in Verona in
Italy over the last 30 years, derived from the local case register, as shown in
Figure 6.1. As the number of psychiatric beds has progressively declined, so the
provision of day care, residential care and out-patient and community contacts
has steadily increased over many years.

While maintenance activities of a newly established system may be less
attractive to innovators, in fact this consolidation is vital to make services
robust and able to survive and thrive in the long term. This will not usually
require a single high-profile leader, but rather a consortium made up of a wider
group of stakeholders who need to co-operate in providing all the service
components within the wider system of care: *'To successfully implement change
in mental health services it is essential to have a shared vision' [New Zealand].*
The successful completion of these policy decisions, and their implementation
on the ground will often also need organised and repeated lobbying by a
coalition of stakeholder groups, to build sufficient political pressure, for
example for modernised mental health laws: *'Meet with policy makers, and
educat[e] them about the Bill, invite them to mental health events, urge them to*

sponsor/co-sponsor the Bill ... and lobby as many legislators as possible to get the Bill passed' [Moldova].

The second overall lesson is that it is essential to: '*Listen to users and families; experiences and perspectives*' [Brazil]. Everyone involved needs to keep a clear focus on the fact that the primary purpose of mental health services is to improve outcomes for people with mental illness. The intended beneficiaries of care therefore need to be – in some sense – in the driving seat when planning and delivering treatment and care. This is a profound transformation, changing from a traditional and paternalistic perspective, in which staff were expected to take all important decisions in the 'best interests' of patients, to an approach in which people with mental illness work, to a far greater extent, in partnership with care providers. This requires a fundamental re-orientation for staff, for example to be and to feel less responsible for deciding all aspects of a patient's life. It also requires that people with mental illness become able to express their views and expectations of care. At the outset this may be very difficult, for example for people who have lived for many years in psychiatric institutions, where their views and preferences were rarely sought or valued. This will often require a stage of support, for example from advocacy workers, so that such individuals can in a sense be re-activated to recognise and express their own points of view. One consequence is that while service quality may improve during a period of developing community mental health services, commonly the expectations of the people being treated rise even faster, leading to a para-doxical decrease in satisfaction. While staff may interpret this as a criticism of the care they provide, another way of looking at this is that such dissatisfaction or complaints are in fact very clear signals of which parts of the service need to be improved next. In other words: '*Service users are the best experts*' [Kyrgyzstan].

The third lesson that emerges from this international consultation is that the team managing such a process needs clear expertise to manage the whole *budget* and that the risks are high that service changes will be used as an occasion for budget cuts: '*Political decision makers need to provide earmarked funding for mental health services, because "soft" services such as mental health are the "underdog" in relation to technologically advanced, high level medical and surgical services*' [Finland]. Having a protected budget is necessary, but not sufficient as it is also vital to be able to exercise flexibility within the overall budget, typically to re-use money saved by reducing the use of in-patient beds for community mental health teams, or occupational or residential services. When such a financial boundary (sometimes called a 'ring fence') for mental health funds is not established and fiercely maintained, then money can easily be diverted to other areas of health care: '*Closing hospital beds makes additional funds available in the global hospital budget!*' [South Africa]. In other words, financial mechanisms need to be created which ensure that: '*Money will follow the patients into the community*' [South Africa].

The next key point is something of a paradox: as mental health care is progressively deinstitutionalised, so some aspects of the mental health system need to be institutionalised! For example, pre-qualification level professional teaching and training curricula will need to be redesigned to include theoretical and practical aspects of delivering care in community settings, and codified in training curricula. Similarly, post-qualifying training courses need to be taught on a regular basis, particularly in the early stages for staff making the transition from hospital to community clinical duties. A further aspect of new forms of institutionalisation is the need for some new legal arrangements; for example, mental health or legal capacity laws may need to be revised or recreated to ensure that their provisions still make sense in the new context, where most clinical contacts between staff and people with mental illnesses take place outside hospitals.

It is clear that the experience base for mental health care can add meaningful information to the ethical and the evidence base. In our view, it is preferable to start with a statement of the principles to guide a new service development (see Chapter 4), and use this in a form of *triangulation* so that the ethical base is combined directly with detailed reviews of the relevant evidence base and experience base to produce the strongest possible case for change.

Key points in this chapter

People committed to better mental health care can expect to face the following key challenges:
- Anxiety and uncertainty in the process of change.
- Need to compensate for a possible lack of structure in community services.
- Uncertainty about how to initiate new developments.
- Deciding how to manage opposition within the mental health system.
- How to deal with opposition from neighbours.
- How to maximise and manage a clearly identified budget.
- Ensuring that rigidities in the old system are made more flexible.
- Creating practical ways to minimise the dysfunctional effects of boundaries between different service components.
- Maintaining staff morale during periods of change.
- Expecting outsiders to know 'what is the right answer?' rather than accepting responsibility for making decisions to suit local circumstances.
The overall key points to bear in mind are that:
- To be improvements that will last, service changes need to take time, and will often be developed over years and decades.

- After the initiation stage of change, often led by charismatic individuals, there will be a necessary consolidation phase.
- Listen to users' and to family members' experiences and perspectives.
- Do not allow service changes to be used as an occasion for budget cuts.
- Consolidate service changes with alterations to training curricula, mental health laws and financial structures.

Acknowledgements

We are grateful for the contribution of the following colleagues: Chantal Van Audenhove and Iris De Coster (Belgium); Cecília Cruz Villares (Brazil); Yiannis Kalakoutas (Cyprus); Kristian Wahlbeck (Finland); Jean Luc Roelandt and Nicolas Daumerie (France); Stefan Weinmann and Thomas Becker (Germany); Nikos Gionakis (Greece); Judit Harangozo (Hungary); Fiona Crowley (Ireland); Roberto Mezzina (Italy); Burul Makenbaeva (Kyrgyzstan); Maris Taube (Latvia); Chee Kok Yoon and Abdul Aziz Abdullah (Malaysia); Sergiu Grozavu (Moldova); Jaap van Weeghel (the Netherlands); Graham Mellsop (New Zealand); Radu Teodorescu (Romania); Pĕtr Nawka (Slovakia); Vesna Švab (Slovenia); Melvyn Freeman and Rita Thom (South Africa); Lars Hansson (Sweden); Ulrich Junghan (Switzerland); Alisher Latypov (Tajikistan); Peykan G. Gökalp (Turkey); Richard Warner (USA).

REFERENCES

1. Box G. *Robustness in Statistics*. London: Academic Press; 1979.
2. Crocker J, Major B and Steele C. Social Stigma. In Gilbert D, Fiske ST and Lindzey G (Eds.). *The Handbook of Social Psychology*, 4th edn. Boston: McGraw-Hill; 1998: 504–533.
3. Thornicroft G. *Shunned: Discrimination against People with Mental Illness*. Oxford: Oxford University Press; 2006.
4. Leff J. *Care in the Community. Illusion or Reality?* London: John Wiley & Sons, Ltd; 1997.
5. Knapp M, Beecham J, Anderson J, *et al.* The TAPS project. 3: Predicting the community costs of closing psychiatric hospitals. *Br. J. Psychiatry* 1990; **157**: 661–670.

7

The geographical dimension: the country/regional level

Defining the country/regional level

This chapter refers to the level at which health policy is formulated, relevant clinical standards are set, and mental health laws are established. Some countries, particularly those with a federal or decentralised political structure, allow regions or states to formulate their own mental health policies. We shall here discuss the key issues relevant at this level for service planning and provision in relation to the social and political, economic and professional domains.

Social and political domains

In the social and political domains, in each country there is a balance to be struck between the concerns of people with mental illness and their families to receive good-quality care, and ensure that their civil liberties are safeguarded, and the legitimate expectations of the wider public that they should be protected from disturbance and harm by people with mental illness, while knowing that proper treatment and care is being provided (see Tables 4.1 and 4.2 in Chapter 4).

In our view it is useful to consider here these key aspects: perceptions of mental illness by the public, by the media, by politicians, and their policy and legal consequences. Although we show this as a linear process in Table 7.1, in fact these are cyclical pathways, and the process can start at any point, although, in our view, public perceptions are often the prime driver of this sequence of perceptions and events.

Within the scheme shown in Table 7.1, mental health policies will reflect the wider mood of the times along a continuum between acceptance and tolerance towards people with mental illness at one extreme, and ignorance, prejudice and discrimination at the other [1]. Regarding tolerance, above all else it seems

Table 7.1 Pathway from social and political perceptions to policy

[A] Perceptions of the Public $\longrightarrow$	[B] Perceptions of Politicians $\longrightarrow$	[C] Policy and Legal Consequences
Influenced by [B], by [C] and by:	Influenced by [A], by [C] and by:	Influenced by [A], by [B] and by:
• Personal experience of mental illness • Family experience • Neighbourhood experiences of services • Word of mouth • Media accounts • Media commentary • Lobbying groups • Professional organisations • Visibility of issues • Social attitudes on civil liberties & public safety • Amount of relevant factual information in the public domain • Attributions on how far people with mental illness are responsible for the conditions	• Personal and family views and experience of politicians • Direct pressure of mass media • Representations of professionals • Mediation of civil servants • Research evidence • Public inquiries • Costs of services • Pressure from other government ministries	• Macro-economic situation • Commercial and business interests • Likelihood of results before the next election • International mental health policies • Influence of international organisations such as World Bank and International Monetary Fund

that direct personal experience of having a mental illness or living with a family member with mental illness is the single most potent factor in encouraging favourable attitudes to these conditions [2–4]. But there remains a powerful paradox: up to three quarters of adults have had such direct experience of mental illness, yet negative reactions to people with mental illness remain the rule [3;5].

The print, broadcast and film media play a complex and very active role in shaping public views about mental illness [6–8]. It is clear that public attitudes *are* changed by strong media messages, which in about two thirds of cases are negative about people with mental illness [9]. In fact the degree of danger from people with mental illness portrayed by the media is grossly disproportionate to any actual risk, and only about 3% of all violent offences are committed by people with mental disorders [10] (see also Thornicroft [1], Chapter 7, for a review of this issue).

Politicians are interpreters of public opinion. They selectively translate their perceptions of the public mood and demands into policy and legal actions. This is a complex process, in which many other factors can be important, such as the personal views and experiences of influential political advisors. At each stage the mediating role of officials and civil servants may also be important, as they offer policy options to elected ministers. Within government, patient-orientated values can often be introduced into policy formulation when clinicians make direct or indirect contributions to the mental health section of the health ministry. Therefore those wishing to make a direct contribution to better mental health care need to establish and maintain very close working relationships with ministers, ministerial advisors, officials and the clinicians involved in formulating and implementing mental health policy at either the regional or the national level [11–13].

To a large extent mental health services more sensitively and subtly reflect the climate of social opinion than most other areas of medical practice. Key concerns include human rights, the position of minority ethnic groups, the problems of marginalised groups, the poor, prisoners and migrants [14;15]. All these issues affect the balance between therapy and control, which will closely reflect wider prevailing public attitudes on how far civil liberties should outweigh risk containment [16].

The economic domain

Economic issues acting at the country level also influence service organisation and development and clinical practice [17;18]. In terms of public expenditure on mental health services, the overall level of economic development (along with the relative importance attached to mental health in relation to other medical specialities) has a profound effect upon the extent and quality of the clinical services available, and upon the capital expenditure available for the construction of health facilities and for their maintenance [14]. The methods used to allocate health expenditure from central finance ministries to local regions, and then to individual local areas, vary enormously, for example in the extent to which these allocation methods take account of local variations in general health or in psychiatric morbidity.

Practically speaking, it is important to realise that mental disorders contribute about 12% of total disability worldwide [19], but in almost all countries the relative investment in mental health is far less than this [20]. In Europe, for example, the average investment is about 5%, with most of this investment spent on in-patient care, and indeed the lowest reported budgets, at less than 2%, are all in the countries of the former Soviet Union [13]. Those advocating for better investment and better services are well advised to brief themselves carefully on the economic arguments before discussing these issues with national or regional governments, for example using these resources [21–25].

The professional domain

The third set of issues acting at the country/regional level are concerns for the professions, including standards of care and agreed staffing levels, training, accreditation and continuing education. *Training* in many countries, for example, is based upon curricula developed when psychiatric services were hospital based. There is often a long delay in which the leading edge of evidence-based clinical practice moves ahead of the content of training courses. Where universities are directly responsible for training and professional education, they need to be both continuously updated of the latest developments in innovative practice and research, and to ensure that their teachers have ongoing active involvement in clinical care and research [26].

One specific way to make such connections is to ensure that as new services develop in community mental health settings, they provide training opportunities for staff. This will mean, for example, that community mental health teams will accept trainee nurses, psychologists, psychiatrists, occupational therapists and social workers so that these posts are a part of the mainstream training curriculum alongside hospital-based training posts.

Further actions which are most often set at the country/regional level are the setting and monitoring of *minimum standards of care*. These may apply to resource issues such as the number of nurses expected to be present on in-patient wards, or the number of doctors for each standard catchment area. National or regional standards can also be set on the content of clinical practice, including the use of agreed prescribing formularies, the adoption of standard diagnostic systems, or the use of evidence-based treatment guidelines and protocols [27;28]. Nevertheless it is clear that current knowledge is more advanced on formulating than on implementing treatment guidelines and protocols [29;30].

Implications

What are the implications of these issues for practical action for better mental health care? Although local details will vary according to the real situation on the ground, the following general steps are likely to be necessary. First, engage in national/regional activities to increase public knowledge about mental illnesses, and to reduce prejudice and discrimination, for example by setting up opportunities for people with mental illness to speak directly to the media about their conditions and their experiences of healthcare. This will involve developing active relationships with those editors and reporters who want to support such changes, and is usually most effectively achieved where the lead is taken by non-governmental service-user and family-member organisations.

Second, in our experience it is vital to have active working relationships with governmental ministers, advisors and civil servants, both in the health and in the social care and finance ministries. Mental health advocacy groups may be more effective if fully informed by research about the frequent occurrence of mental illness [31], the cost implications of these conditions, and the latest evidence of effective treatments. These high-level policy contacts then need to be used for organised and relentless advocacy by the mental health sector to increase investment in mental healthcare.

Third, in the longer term there is a need to ensure that the training curricula for all mental health care professionals and practitioners are continuously revised to take account of the latest clinical developments and research findings. At the same time, as community mental health services develop they need to include training posts for all the relevant disciplines.

Key points in this chapter

- The country/regional level refers to the level at which health policy is formulated, relevant clinical standards are set, and mental health laws are established.
- At country/regional level an interplay between the perceptions of the public and of politicians has an important bearing on how far mental health laws and policies are liberal or restrictive.
- Although mental disorders contribute about 12% of total disability worldwide, in almost all countries the relative investment in mental health is far less than this.
- An important activity at the country/regional level is the setting and monitoring of minimum standards of care.
- There is a need to ensure that the training curricula for mental health practitioners are continuously revised to take account of the latest clinical developments and research findings.

REFERENCES

1. Thornicroft G. *Shunned: Discrimination Against People with Mental Illness.* Oxford: Oxford University Press; 2006.
2. Crisp AH, Cowan L and Hart D. The College's anti-stigma campaign 1998–2003. *Psychiatr. Bull.* 2004; **28**: 133–136.
3. Pinfold V, Thornicroft G, Huxley P and Farmer P. Active ingredients in anti-stigma programmes in mental health. *Int. Rev. Psychiatry* 2005; **17**(2): 123–131.
4. Corrigan P. *On the Stigma of Mental Illness.* Washington, DC: American Psychological Association; 2005.

5. Crisp A, Gelder MG, Goddard E and Meltzer H. Stigmatization of people with mental illnesses: a follow-up study within the Changing Minds campaign of the Royal College of Psychiatrists. *World Psychiatry* 2005; **4**: 106–113.

6. Wahl OF. *Media Madness: Public Images of Mental Illness.* New Brunswick, NJ: Rutgers University Press; 1995.

7. Angermeyer MC, Dietrich S, Pott D and Matschinger H. Media consumption and desire for social distance towards people with schizophrenia. *Eur. Psychiatry* 2005; **20**(3): 246–250.

8. Nairn RG and Coverdale JH. People never see us living well: an appraisal of the personal stories about mental illness in a prospective print media sample. *Aust. N. Z. J. Psychiatry* 2005; **39**(4): 281–287.

9. Angermeyer MC and Matschinger H. Have there been any changes in the public's attitudes towards psychiatric treatment? Results from representative population surveys in Germany in the years 1990 and 2001. *Acta Psychiatr. Scand.* 2005; **111**(1): 68–73.

10. Swanson JW. Mental disorder, substance abuse, and community violence: An epidemiological approach. In Monahan J and Steadman HJ (Eds.). *Violence and Mental Disorder.* Chicago: University of Chicago Press; 1994. 101–136.

11. World Health Organisation. *WHO Resource Book on Mental Health, Human Rights and Legislation.* Geneva: World Health Organisation; 2005.

12. World Health Organisation. World Health Report 2001. *Mental Health: New Understanding, New Hope.* Geneva: World Health Organization; 2001.

13. Knapp MJ, McDaid D, Mossialos E and Thornicroft G. *Mental Health Policy and Practice Across Europe.* Buckingham: Open University Press; 2006.

14. Patel V, Saraceno B and Kleinman A. Beyond evidence: the moral case for international mental health. *Am. J. Psychiatry* 2006; **163**(8): 1312–1315.

15. Desjarlais R, Eisenberg L, Good B and Kleinman A. *World Mental Health. Problems and Priorities in Low Income Countries.* Oxford: Oxford University Press; 1995.

16. Furedi F. *Culture of Fear: Risk Taking and the Morality of Low Expectations.* London: Cassell Academic; 1997.

17. Knapp M. *The Economic Evaluation of Mental Health Care.* London: Arena; 1995.

18. Frank RG and Manning WG (Eds). *Economics and Mental Health.* Baltimore: Johns Hopkins University Press; 1992.

19. Murray C and Lopez A. *The Global Burden of Disease, Vol. 1. A Comprehensive Assessment of Mortality and Disability from Diseases, Injuries and Risk Factors in 1990, and Projected to 2020.* Cambridge, MA: Harvard University Press; 1996.

20. World Health Organisation. *Investing in Mental Health.* Geneva: World Health Organisation; 2003.

21. World Health Organization. *Advocacy for Mental Health.* Geneva: World Health Organization; 2003.

22. World Health Organisation. *Mental Health Financing.* Geneva: World Health Organisation; 2003.

23. World Health Organisation. *Mental Health Policy, Plans and Programmes.* Geneva: World Health Organization; 2004.

24. World Health Organisation. *Planning and Budgeting to Deliver Services for Mental Health.* Geneva: World Health Organization; 2003.

25. Warner R. *Recovery from Schizophrenia: Psychiatry and Political Economy*. Hove: Brunner-Routledge; 2004.

26. Lader EW, Cannon CP, Ohman EM, *et al.* The clinician as investigator: participating in clinical trials in the practice setting. *Circulation* 2004; **109**(21): 2672–2679.

27. Torrey WC, Drake RE, Dixon L, *et al.* Implementing evidence-based practices for persons with severe mental illnesses. *Psychiatr. Serv.* 2001; **52**(1): 45–50.

28. Wells K, Miranda J, Bruce ML, Alegria M and Wallerstein N. Bridging community intervention and mental health services research. *Am. J. Psychiatry* 2004; **161**(6): 955–963.

29. Wells K, Sherbourne C, Schoenbaum M, *et al.* Five-year impact of quality improvement for depression: results of a group-level randomized controlled trial. *Arch. Gen. Psychiatry* 2004; **61**(4): 378–386.

30. Drake RE, Goldman HH, Leff HS, *et al.* Implementing evidence-based practices in routine mental health service settings. *Psychiatr. Serv.* 2001; **52**(2): 179–182.

31. Kessler RC, Demler O, Frank RG, *et al.* Prevalence and treatment of mental disorders, 1990 to 2003. *N. Engl. J. Med. 2005*; **352**(24): 2515–2523.

8

The geographical dimension: the local level

Defining the local level

The local level may be seen as intermediate between the national/regional and the individual levels. The basis for defining the boundary of this level will vary considerably between different places. In some countries there will be a clear geographical basis to define the local level, for example an area of perhaps 250000–500000 population which is served by a single health organisation or for whom services are commissioned by a single funding agency. In other areas there may be sectoral arrangements on the basis of eligibility, for example the Veterans Administration provides healthcare for military personnel in the USA, and in this case the overall pattern of care consists of overlapping local levels of service from different care providers.

Even within relatively integrated public-service systems, there may be different boundaries for local primary health care, specialist mental health care and social-services provision. Indeed, in some countries (such as the UK) such importance is attached to primary care that local specialist services (such as mental health care) are defined by the lists of patients registered by groups of local family doctors [1].

Where a greater emphasis is put upon patients as consumers, then increasingly policy-makers stress that it is important to allow choices in services from a mixed economy of providers, and this adds greater complexity to the simple idea of integrated local care in geographical terms.

Service functions at the local level

Where local services are organised on the basis of population catchment areas at the local level, these are often called sectors. The concept of the sector has permeated community mental health service development. Following the emergence of the first sectors in France in 1947, by 1961 over 300 had been

Table 8.1 Factors influencing the scale of a general adult mental health service

Factors in the population

(1) Socio-demographic composition
(2) Social deprivation
(3) Ethnic composition
(4) Age–sex structure
(5) Psychiatric morbidity
(6) Existing patterns of service use
(7) Population density

Factors in the local area

(1) Significant geographical features
(2) Degree of urbanicity

Factors in the organisation of services

(1) Social services boundaries
(2) Primary care organisation
(3) Historical patient referral patterns

established. In the USA the Community Mental Health Centres Act (1963) introduced the principle of a catchment area for each CMHC, and by 1975, 40% of the population had sectorised services [2;3]. A further range of factors can also affect the choice of sector scale and they are shown in Table 8.1.

Over the last decade there has been a trend away from a population catchment area basis for providing sectorised care, and towards a functional view of local services. This reflects both the practical consequences of allowing greater choice for service-users, and the growing tendency for governments (including those whose national health services formerly had a monopoly in providing care) to see their primary role in commissioning or regulating services, and encouraging a market-orientated, mixed economy of state, for profit and non-governmental organisations to provide treatment and care services [4].

It may now be clearer to consider local services in functional terms, in which the overall system, and its component services, are understood in terms of the core activities and functions that they provide. Within a general adult mental health service (see Chapter 5) typically these functions are provided by the five key components: out-patient/ambulatory clinics, community mental health teams [5], acute in-patient care, long-term community-based residential care [6], and rehabilitation, occupation and work. These core functions are usually delivered to smaller populations than the highly specialised teams (such as specialist out-patient clinics for people with eating disorders, dual diagnosis, treatment-resistant affective disorders, adolescent; or for specialised mobile mental health teams such as assertive community treatment teams or home treatment teams [7;8]), see Table 5.4 [9].

Table 8.2 Advantages of organising services at the local level

Planning Advantages

(1) High identification of rates of patients
(2) Feasible scale for clinical and social assessments
(3) Assists the integration of local service components
(4) Greater budgetary clarity for defined population

Service delivery advantages

(1) Minimises patients lost to follow up
(2) Facilitates home treatment
(3) Improved identity of staff with local population
(4) Facilitates inter-agency collaboration
(5) Provides population denominator for research and evaluation

Quality of service advantages

(1) Less use of crisis and in-patient facilities
(2) Improved patient education and intervention
(3) Greater support of relatives and carers
(4) Defined responsibility for each patient
(5) Improved communication for staff, patients and carers
(6) Improved primary–secondary service communication

One important feature of community-orientated services is their accessibility to people with mental illnesses (see Tables 4.2 and 4.5). For service fixed to a static site, such as in-patient units, it is important that they are reasonably accessible to those whom they service, for example in terms of distance and travelling time. For mobile service components, such as community mental health teams, these are essentially locally defined by virtue of the territory which they can effectively cover to visit people with mental illness at home [10]. There is a series of additional advantages to locally provided mental health care, as summarised in Table 8.2.

Engagement with local stakeholders

Working at the local level makes building links with key local figures in the local community both necessary and useful. They will most often include, not only family doctors, general hospital and other health service clinicians, but also the whole range of interests shown in Table 8.3. But a wider array of stakeholders may also wish to have their interests represented and taken into account in decision-making. These constituencies may include: neighbourhood or residents' associations, local school staff, governors and parents, representatives of different cultural and ethnic communities, shopkeepers and members of local

Table 8.3 Key stakeholders at the local level

- Service-users/consumers
- Family members/carers
- Health care professionals (mental health and primary care staff)
- Other public services agencies e.g. police and housing
- Other service-provider groups, e.g. non-governmental organisations, church and charitable groups
- Policy-makers: politicians, political advisers and officials
- Service planners and commissioners
- Advocacy groups
- Local media, e.g. newspaper and radio

business, and church ministers and elders of other faith communities. The importance of these stakeholders emerges particularly at times when plans are being developed to open new mental health facilities, and meaningful consultations at this stage may prevent local opposition which could stop community services from being initiated.

Implications of focusing on the local level

Our emphasis on the primacy of the local level within the geographical dimension leads us to make explicit that the work of mental health services is more similar to primary care than most other specialist health services. This is so because what they have in common is not only a responsibility for a given (and usually geographically defined) patient population, but also a longitudinal perspective in assessing and treating patients (which hospital specialists with a typically cross-sectional or episodic approach will not be able to develop). Moreover, they will both adopt a clinical perspective which regards treatment and rehabilitation as a continuum rather than as conceptually and practically distinct. As some other areas of medicine, such as rheumatology, metabolic diseases or geriatrics, develop systems of service for patients with chronic or relapsing and remitting conditions, we expect that these skills will become more widespread in future.

On a more cautious note, in some particular areas the local level, as we conceptualise it here, may not exist in terms of the organisation of services. Most European countries have an administrative infrastructure which organises health, social and other public services for defined geographical areas. On the other hand, health systems with a greater degree of deregulation, such as those in most parts of the United States, may only weakly reflect the public health approach, without which a meaningful and efficient integration of services, which we consider to be the central purpose of the local level, becomes extremely difficult to achieve. For the reasons given in this chapter, we are drawn to the conclusion that *locality* is the central organising theme for the efficient planning, organisation and delivery of mental health treatment and care.

Key points in this chapter

- Where local services are organised on the basis of population catchment areas at the local level, these are often called sectors, typically serving 50000–80000 total population.
- A general adult mental health service typically includes five key functions: out-patient/ambulatory clinics, community mental health teams, acute in-patient care, long-term community-based residential care, and rehabilitation, occupation and work.
- Developing local services is often best done in close collaboration with a range of local stakeholders including: service-users, family members, advocacy groups, health care staff, other public services agencies, e.g. police and housing, non-governmental organisations, church and charitable groups, policy-makers: politicians, political advisers, and officials, and service planners and commissioners

REFERENCES

1. Olson RP. *Mental Health Systems Compared: Great Britain, Norway, Canada and the United States.* Springfield, IL: Charles C. Thomas; 2006.
2. Grob G. *From Asylum to Community. Mental Health Policy in Modern America.* Princeton, NJ: Princeton University Press; 1991.
3. Hansson L. Sectorization. In Thornicroft G and Szmukler G (Eds.). *Textbook of Community Psychiatry.* Oxford: Oxford University Press; 2001: 215–222.
4. Knapp MJ, McDaid D, Mossialos E and Thornicroft G. *Mental Health Policy and Practice Across Europe.* Buckingham: Open University Press; 2006.
5. Burns T. *Community Mental Health Teams: A Guide to Current Practices.* Oxford: Oxford University Press; 2004.
6. Leff JP. *Care in the Community: Illusion or reality?* Chichester: John Wiley & Sons, Ltd; 2003.
7. Killaspy H, Bebbington P, Blizard R, *et al.* The REACT study: randomised evaluation of assertive community treatment in north London. *BMJ* 2006; **332**(7545): 815–820.
8. Johnson S, Nolan F, Pilling S, *et al.* Randomised controlled trial of acute mental health care by a crisis resolution team: the north Islington crisis study. *BMJ* 2005; **331**(7517): 599.
9. Thornicroft G and Szmukler G. *Textbook of Community Psychiatry.* Oxford: Oxford University Press; 2001.
10. Burns T, Knapp M, Catty J, *et al.* Home treatment for mental health problems: a systematic review. *Health Technol. Assess* 2003 **5**,15.

The geographical dimension: the individual level

Defining the individual level

By the individual level we refer to the level for interventions for individual service-users, and their family members, as well as their immediate social networks. This level is traditionally considered to be the proper territory of the clinician or practitioner, but as we shall argue in the next two chapters, the outcome of care also strongly depends upon the characteristics of the other two geographical levels (local and national). It is therefore important for clinicians to be aware of how processes at these higher levels can positively or negatively influence their direct clinical work.

The significance of the individual level

At this level, we wish to emphasise three points: (i) the research evidence in the field of mental health is mainly concentrated at the individual level more than at the local level (see Chapter 10), often from samples that are not fully representative of the wider populations of people with mental illness; (ii) the evidence base generally applies to single clinical interventions rather than to treatment combinations and (iii) whatever the evidence base, often there is not a close correspondence between what the evidence suggests as effective interventions and actual clinical practice [1;2]. This can go in both directions. Effective practice may be in advance of, or lag behind, the latest evidence base. From this it is clear that both directions need to be used as methods of learning how to improve care. Further, it is important to appreciate that a lack of evidence about a particular intervention is not the same as evidence for its lack of effectiveness. An unevaluated treatment, for example, may or may not be effective.

In traditional clinical practice, doctors see the individuals who come to their attention and they base their views on the likely outcome upon their accumulating direct clinical experience, which mostly concerns people with mental

Table 9.1 Key elements for interventions at the individual level

- Seeing the individual as a partner in treatment
- Recognising the whole range of needs for each individual
- Using the individual's family members and carers as a resource

illness. The clinician's illusion, as it has been called [3], means that most people who improve and recover leave care, and therefore over time a practitioner's experience is more and more of treating people with long-term conditions, so that they tend to base their views about prognosis upon their own unrepresentative experience of treating people with a poorer than average outcome. For these understandable reasons they may give over-pessimistic advice to people with mental illness and their families [3–5]. What are the most important issues at the individual level? We have identified three key elements which we now discuss in turn in this chapter, as shown in Table 9.1.

Seeing the individual as a partner in care

The first step in establishing a therapeutic relationship between clinician and individual is to try to develop a partnership in which both work together to identify the problems to be tackled and jointly to agree a care plan [6;7]. Put differently this can be seen as practitioners offering the type of care that they would like to receive if the roles were exchanged [8]. Such relationships have been described as falling under three headings: the paternalistic model, where the doctor decides what to do; the informed model, in which the patient decides after the doctor explains the options; and the shared model, where doctor and patient decide together what action to take. Indeed the editor of the *BMJ* has expressed the view that 'moving to the shared model may be the most important change in medicine in the next decade.' [9].

When individuals are informed in this way, it becomes possible to see them as *negotiators* in their own treatment. This negotiating position applies equally to psychological and social types of treatment, such as participation at a day centre or in applying for work. In relation to medication, it is important to realise that for many physical and mental disorders, individuals in fact only take their medication as prescribed about half the time [10]. For example, people with psychotic conditions who have experienced adverse effects of anti-psychotic medication, and who may therefore be understandably reluctant to take more, may wish to agree with their doctor a dose range within which the individual has day-to-day discretion over the dose taken. Such preferences can be expressed within an advance directive or crisis plan [11;12].

Such a negotiating stance is pragmatic since, in our own clinical experience, it is likely to increase the likelihood of individuals acting upon a recommended medication regime or treatment plan. But there are also wider ethical reasons for such a partnership approach. Recent research in the USA indicates that individuals' perceptions of coercion during in-patient treatment are less when they report that they: (i) have had an opportunity at some time during the admission to give a full account from their own point of view of the admission and (ii) have felt that their account has been taken seriously by staff. These two factors are referred to by the MacArthur Network researchers as 'procedural justice', and indicate that when individuals report that they have been treated respectfully in these two particular ways, they consequently find their treatment more acceptable, even if the admission has been compulsory, or if they have received enforced medication at some stage during their in-patient treatment [13–15].

Indeed, this approach is already common for some types of treatment, for example certain forms of psychotherapy, especially behavioural and cognitive-behavioural treatments, have made explicit and have systematised such active individual participation. Related to this, it is important to emphasise that we propose negotiating primarily about treatments of *established and known effectiveness*, so that individual participation in care decisions can be seen as both principled and pragmatic.

Recognising the whole range of individual needs

Staff in modern mental health care practice need to consider a wide range of biological, psychological and social needs. It has become clear in recent years that an individual's view of his or her own needs and the view of the practitioner may be substantially different [16–18]. Indeed service-user-rated needs are much better predictors of quality of life than are staff-rated needs [19]. Interestingly, where staff and service-user ratings of need do agree closely, then this predicts a better long-term outcome of care [20]. A method which can be used to assess the whole range of needs is provided by the Camberwell Assessment of Need (CAN) [21;22] (see Table 9.2).

Using the individual's family members and carers as a resource

The family members and carers of a person with mental illness are often a valuable resource to work with mental health staff [23]. Specific techniques for working with such families and methods of measuring their involvement and the impact of caring have received attention in the literature [24]. To realise the potential for family members to play a full role in planning and providing care,

Table 9.2 Areas of need included in Camberwell Assessment of Need (CAN)

- Accommodation
- Occupation
- Specific psychotic symptoms
- Psychological distress
- Information about condition and treatment
- Non-prescribed drugs
- Food and meals
- Household skills
- Self care and presentation
- Safety to self
- Safety to others
- Money
- Childcare
- Physical health
- Alcohol
- Basic education
- Company
- Telephone
- Public transport
- Welfare benefits

their own concerns need to be understood, and their own direct needs addressed. One example of this recognition is Standard 6 of the National Service Framework for Mental Health in England which is called 'Caring about Carers' [25]. This requires all individuals who provide regular and substantial care for a person with severe mental illness to have an annual assessment of their own needs, and to have their own care plan to assist them in their care-giving role. What are the common concerns of family members? These are shown in Table 9.3 [26].

In fact, staff may unintentionally exclude family members from playing a full role in caring, for example by 'confidentiality' to prevent communication. Carers often report that their attempts to talk to staff are frustrated by hearing that they cannot be brought into discussions about their relative's care for reasons of confidentiality [27], that is, clinical information is not disclosed to third parties without the consent of the person concerned. While this is a legal requirement in many countries, staff often fail to recognise that relatives cannot act on an informed basis to support the person if they are specifically excluded from access to the relevant facts. One way to reconcile these apparently contradictory needs is for clinicians to raise this issue explicitly with the service-user to gain authorisation about what information can be shared with which family member [28]. A less formal, but often more helpful, way to involve family

Table 9.3 Common concerns of family members of people with mental illness

- Loss of the expected future of the person with mental illness
- Worry about suicide and aggressive behaviour
- Concern about underactivity by their unwell relative
- Need for information on the condition, its treatment and implications
- Information on whether family actions or neglect have caused the disorder
- Expert advice about welfare benefit entitlements
- Effects on the mental health of other family members
- Need for periods of respite
- What will happen in future when the family member/carer dies

members is to invite them to attend clinical appointments at which both the family and the individual are present. At the very minimum, even if the person with mental illness has not given permission for clinical information to be conveyed to relatives, then staff can still listen to what family members wish to say, which very often contains very important information about the condition of the person with mental illness. In other words, staff are rarely justified in completely excluding family members from care-planning discussions.

Not too much and not too little care

While institutions provide 'total care' to people cared for within their confines, one important advantage of community-orientated care is that the degree of assistance provided to people with mental illness can be titrated to their current needs. Yet with a balance of hospital and community-care provision, in many of the more economically developed countries, most individuals with mental illness will never seek help. Even when people do go to a doctor, for example, for mental helath problems, this may be after very long periods of delay or avoidance of treatment services. People with social phobia, for example, can wait, on average, for up to 14 years before contacting mental health services [29]. Practitioners can therefore indirectly assist individuals by measures which encourage help-seeking, for example by taking part in effective public education or anti-stigma activities [30;31]. Related to this, steps to detect developing mental illnesses and to provide treatment at an early stage may be vital to reduce the long-term and potentially disabling consequences of the condition [32;33], using the following guidelines:

- Encouraging people to seek help
- Active early detection of developing mental illness
- Service-user empowerment to plan for recovery and to identify relapses early
- Provide flexible support according to current needs

- Provide reliable and rapid crisis response when necessary
- Supported risk-taking to manageable demands and reduce unnecessary dependence.

As many forms of mental illness can follow a so-called 'remitting and relapsing' pattern, in which the person with mental illness has periods of relative recovery between episodes of being unwell, methods developed for other similar conditions (for example, rheumatoid arthritis) may also be applicable. Some of these recent approaches are called 'disease management' or 'condition management' programmes [34;35]. A critical ingredient is the provision of sufficient information to the service-user to allow the person to make informed choices about treatment options [36;37]. A further active ingredient necessary for health care professions to accept is that the person affected by the illness has control over which treatments to accept and which to reject or defer: in other words, an empowerment approach [38]. From this viewpoint, in relation to conditions such as bipolar disorder, schizophrenia and recurrent depression, the clinician can be ready to provide higher or lower levels of treatment according to the changing needs of the person: so that not too little, but also not too much input is provided. The risk is that the over-provision of treatment and care can lead to a long-term dependency and a progressive loss of autonomy and empowerment.

The over-provision of treatment or care may mean, for example, continuing an unnecessarily high dosage of an anti-psychotic medication when the person's condition has already substantially improved; or it may mean a prolonged period of in-patient treatment, which can lead to the loss of everyday living skills and to progressive institutionalisation.

As clear-cut markers to indicate the beginning of an episode of mental illness do not currently exist, practitioners and service-users need to use their experience and judgement to assess early signs of illness. In this respect service-users (and their family members) are often in a much better position to detect the very earliest features of a relapse than are practitioners. In the same way, signs of recovery need to be equally recognised as early as possible, to alert staff to reduce the degree of intervention and to allow a progressively greater degree of empowerment and return to everyday life (for example in reducing medication doses, or in less frequent appointments).

Even so, during a period of recovery there are difficult decisions to take about how much stress is manageable for the person, for example, when to return to work and whether to take part-time duties, and at what stages this may promote further recovery or, in fact, lead to a prompt relapse. For the best of reasons, staff and family members may continue to be protective for longer than is necessary.

There is very little research evidence about how much stress is advisable at what stage of recovery, and so usually these decisions depend upon difficult judgements. One approach is to avoid stressful life events to minimise the likelihood of relapse, but, in this case, the person is protected both from such stressors and from the possibility of successfully returning to his or her normal life. An approach favoured by many service-user and consumer-advocacy groups is self-management, in which stepped risks, such as a return to work, are taken with strong family and professional support [39]. This is the supported risk-taking perspective, with the key decisions taken by the service-user. One of the most important supports that is often needed is confidence by the person with mental illness and family members that if the person has a crisis, that they will be able to gain access to expert help very quickly.

Further, in relation to timing, good clinical practice demonstrates the capacity to provide services that can both rapidly increase and rapidly decrease in intensity according to the condition of the individual. Often, however, it is the case that services are simply unable to respond in a timely fashion at all, or are only able to increase their input quickly, but are slow to withdraw the amount of care during the individual's recovery.

Key points in this chapter

- By the individual level we refer to the level for interventions for individual service users, and their family members, as well as their immediate social networks.
- The research evidence in the field of mental health is mainly concentrated at the individual level more than at the local level.
- The evidence base generally applies to single clinical interventions rather than to treatment combinations.
- There is often not a close correspondence between what the evidence suggests as effective interventions and actual clinical practice.
- Because practitioners often spend more time with those people whose mental illnesses have the poorest outcomes, such staff can develop an unjustified pessimism about the prognosis for mental illnesses.
- We support the view that service-users be seen as 'partners in care' so that treatment plans are negotiated, and family members fully involved in care.
- The recovery approach, stressing optimism for the future, is one that is gaining support in many countries.

REFERENCES

1. Geddes JR and Harrison PJ. Closing the gap between research and practice. *Br. J. Psychiatry* 1997; **171**: 220–225.
2. Tansella M, Thornicroft G, Barbui C, Cipriani A and Saraceno B. Seven criteria to improve effectiveness trials in psychiatry. *Psychol. Med.* (in press) 2006; **36**(5): 711–720.

3. Cohen P and Cohen J. The clinician's illusion. *Arch. Gen. Psychiatry.* 1984; **41**(12): 1178–1182.

4. Vessey JT, Howard KI, Lueger RJ, Kachele H and Mergenthaler E. The clinician's illusion and the psychotherapy practice: an application of stochastic modeling. *J. Consult. Clin. Psychol.* 1994; **62**(4): 679–685.

5. Phelan JC, Yang LH and Cruz-Rojas R. Effects of attributing serious mental illnesses to genetic causes on orientations to treatment. *Psychiatr. Serv.* 2006; **57**(3): 382–387.

6. Haigh R. Partnership with patients. Modern antipaternalism needs to be invigorated. *BMJ* 2000; **320**(7227): 117–118.

7. Coulter A. Paternalism or partnership? *BMJ* 1999; **319**: 719–720.

8. Bleker OP. Partnership with patients. Treat patients as you would like to be treated yourself. *BMJ* 2000; **320**(7227): 117.

9. Smith R. Take your partners for the dance. *BMJ* 1999; **319**(7212): A.

10. Haynes RB, McDonald HP and Garg AX. *Interventions For Helping Patients to Follow Prescriptions For Medications.* Oxford: Cochrane Library Update Software Issue 2; 2002.

11. Henderson C, Flood C, Leese M, *et al.* Effect of joint crisis plans on use of compulsory treatment in psychiatry: single blind randomised controlled trial. *BMJ* 2004; **329**(7458): 136.

12. Flood C, Byford S, Henderson C, *et al.* Joint crisis plans for people with psychosis: economic evaluation of a randomised controlled trial. *BMJ* 2006; **333**(7571): 729.

13. Szmukler G and Appelbaum P. Treatment pressures, coercion and compulsion. In Thornicroft G and Szmukler G (Eds.). *Textbook of Community Psychiatry.* Oxford: Oxford University Press; 2001: 529–544.

14. Elbogen EB, Swanson JW and Swartz MS. Effects of legal mechanisms on perceived coercion and treatment adherence among persons with severe mental illness. *J. Nerv. Ment. Dis.* 2003; **191**(10): 629–637.

15. Bindman J, Reid Y, Szmukler G, *et al.* Perceived coercion at admission to psychiatric hospital and engagement with follow-up: a cohort study. *Soc. Psychiatry Psychiatr. Epidemiol.* 2005; **40**(2): 160–166.

16. Lasalvia A, Ruggeri M, Mazzi MA and Dall'Agnola RB. The perception of needs for care in staff and patients in community-based mental health services. The South-Verona Outcome Project 3. *Acta Psychiatr. Scand.* 2000; **102**(5): 366–375.

17. Lasalvia A, Bonetto C, Malchiodi F, *et al.* Listening to patients' needs to improve their subjective quality of life. *Psychol. Med.* 2005; **35**(11): 1655–1665.

18. Thornicroft G and Slade M. Comparing needs assessed by staff and by service users: paternalism or partnership in mental health? *Epidemiol. Psichiatr. Soc.* 2002; **11**(3): 186–191.

19. Slade M, Leese M, Cahill S, Thornicroft G and Kuipers E. Patient-rated mental health needs and quality of life improvement. *Br. J. Psychiatry* 2005; **187**: 256–261.

20. Lasalvia A and Ruggeri M. Multidimensional outcomes in 'real world' mental health services: follow-up findings from the South Verona Project. *Acta Psychiatr. Scand. (Suppl.)* 2007; **116**: 3–77.

21. Slade M, Thornicroft G, Loftus L, Phelan M and Wykes T. *CAN: The Camberwell Assessment of Need.* London: Gaskell, Royal College of Psychiatrists; 1999.

22. Thomas S, Harty M, Parrott J, *et al. The Forensic CAN: A Needs Assessment For Forensic Mental Health Service Users*. London: Gaskell, Royal College of Psychiatrists; 2003.

23. Mueser KT and Gingerich S. *Coping with Schizophrenia: A Guide for Families*. New York: Guildford Press; 2005.

24. Joyce J, Leese M, Kuipers E, *et al*. Evaluating a model of caregiving for people with psychosis. *Soc. Psychiatry Psychiatr. Epidemiol*. 2003; **38**(4): 189–195.

25. Department of Health. *National Service Framework for Mental Health. Modern Standards and Service Models*. London: Department of Health; 1999.

26. Berry D, Szmukler G and Thornicroft G. *Living with Schizophrenia: The Carers Story*. Brighton: Pavillion Press; 1997.

27. Rapaport J, Bellringer S, Pinfold V and Huxley P. Carers and confidentiality in mental health care: considering the role of the carer's assessment. A study of service users', carers' and practitioners' views. *Health Soc. Care Community* 2006; **14**(4): 357–365.

28. Szmukler GI and Bloch S. Family involvement in the care of people with psychoses. An ethical argument. *Br. J. Psychiatry* 1997; **171**: 401–405.

29. Dingemans AE, Couvee J and Westenberg HG. Characteristics of patients with social phobia and their treatment in specialized clinics for anxiety disorders in the Netherlands. *J. Affect. Disord*. 2001; **65**(2): 123–129.

30. Griffiths KM, Christensen H, Jorm AF, Evans K and Groves C. Effect of web-based depression literacy and cognitive-behavioural therapy interventions on stigmatising attitudes to depression: randomised controlled trial. *Br. J. Psychiatry* 2004; **185**: 342–349.

31. Thornicroft G. *Shunned: Discrimination Against People With Mental Illness*. Oxford: Oxford University Press; 2006.

32. Perkins DO, Gu H, Boteva K and Lieberman JA. Relationship between duration of untreated psychosis and outcome in first-episode schizophrenia: a critical review and meta-analysis. *Am. J. Psychiatry* 2005; **162**(10): 1785–1804.

33. Friis S, Vaglum P, Haahr U, *et al*. Effect of an early detection programme on duration of untreated psychosis: part of the Scandinavian TIPS study. *Br. J. Psychiatry Suppl*. 2005; **48**: s29-s32.

34. Warsi A, Wang PS, LaValley MP, Avorn J and Solomon DH. Self-management education programs in chronic disease: a systematic review and methodological critique of the literature. *Arch. Intern. Med*. 2004; **164**(15): 1641–1649.

35. Ofman JJ, Badamgarav E, Henning JM, *et al*. Does disease management improve clinical and economic outcomes in patients with chronic diseases? A systematic review. *Am. J. Med*. 2004; **117**(3): 182–192.

36. Harris M, Smith B and Veale A. Printed patient education interventions to facilitate shared management of chronic disease: a literature review. *Intern. Med. J*. 2005; **35**(12): 711–716.

37. Mueser KT, Corrigan PW, Hilton DW, *et al*. Illness management and recovery: a review of the research. *Psychiatr. Serv*. 2002; **53**(10): 1272–1284.

38. Corrigan PW. Empowerment and serious mental illness: treatment partnerships and community opportunities. *Psychiatr. Q*. 2002; **73**(3): 217–228.

39. Chamberlin J. User/consumer involvement in mental health service delivery. *Epidemiol. Psychiatr. Soc*. 2005.

10

The time dimension: the input phase

Defining the input phase

Inputs are those resources which are introduced into the mental health system, and which need to be distinguished from the *processes* which take place within that system, which we describe in the next chapter. These inputs can be introduced into the mental health system at the three geographical levels, and may also be described as either visible or invisible.

Visible inputs consist mainly of staff and buildings. In psychiatry, compared with other medical specialities, relatively little is spent on equipment, as most expenditure is on staff costs, which include the salaries of nurses, psychiatrists, psychologists, social workers and other practitioners.

Sometimes forgotten are the *invisible inputs*, such as good working relationships. These are often ignored or undervalued, even though they can enhance or inhibit the effects of visible inputs. Indeed the influence of such invisible inputs often only becomes manifest when they are absent. Without good working relationships, for example, referrals of cases between teams can be blocked or delayed, reducing the quality of care. Other invisible inputs include staff experience and expertise. Recently this has been increasingly recognised by assessing treatment fidelity, namely how far staff interventions adhere to evidence-based standards.

In our view, the primary purpose of a mental health service should be to deliver effective interventions to individuals with mental illness (cell 3C of the matrix model in Table 10.2). Therefore inputs are *only* worthwhile if they contribute directly or indirectly towards improved outcomes for individuals. Even so, financial inputs, which are relatively easy to quantify, are often used as indicators of system performance. Indeed, it is common for governments to describe increased expenditure on mental health services *as if* this is identical to providing a better service. It is not. The vital point is whether inputs contribute towards measurable and improved outcomes.

Table 10.1 Categories of input to mental health services

VISIBLE INPUTS

- **Budget**
  - ○ Absolute amount of monetary resources allocated to mental health services
  - ○ Relative allocation in comparison with total health expenditure

- **Staff**
  - ○ Numbers of staff in relation to population served
  - ○ Mix of professions and seniority grades

- **Buildings, facilities and equipment**

- **Equipment for investigation, diagnosis and treatment**

INVISIBLE INPUTS

- **Working relationships**
  - ○ Between staff within clinical teams
  - ○ Between different clinical mental health teams
  - ○ Between mental health and physical health teams

- **Policies and regulations**
  - ○ Mental health and related laws
  - ○ Organisational policies and quality standards
  - ○ Treatment protocols and guidelines

- **Public stigma and media representations of mental illness**

In this chapter we shall illustrate inputs in relation to the main categories of mental health care, as shown in Table 10.1, and we shall discuss these in relation to the three geographical levels, as illustrated in Table 10.2.

Inputs at the country/regional level

In terms of *budget allocations*, there are huge variations between countries (and between regions within countries) in their actual financial allocations for mental health care. WHO estimates that 12% of the total global burden of disease (GBD) can be attributed to psychiatric disorders. GBD takes into account both mortality (years of life lost, YLL) and morbidity (disability adjusted life years, DALY). For mortality, for example, each year a reported 800 000 people commit suicide worldwide, 86% in low- and middle-income countries, most involving people aged 15–44. In relation to disability, in 2002 32% of global DALYs were caused by mental disorders – the leading contributor to GBD among the non-communicable diseases (NCD), more than cardiovascular disease (22% of NCD DALYs) or cancer (11%). In the UK the costs of providing medical and social care for people with dementia alone are greater than cancer and cardiovascular disease combined. By comparison,

Table 10.2 Overview of the matrix model, with key issues at the input phase

Place Dimension	Time Dimension		
	(A) Input phase	(B) Process phase	(C) Outcome phase
(1) Country/ regional level	1A • Mental health budget allocation • Mental health laws • Government directives and policies • Training plans for mental health staff • Treatment protocols and guidelines	1B	1C
(2) Local level	2A • Local service budgets and balance for hospital and community services • Local population needs assessment • Staff numbers and mix • Clinical and non-clinical services • Working relationships between teams	2B	2C
(3) Individual level	3A • Assessments of individual needs made by staff, service users and by families • Therapeutic expertise of staff • Information for service users • Information for family members	3B	3C

only 2% of all health budgets worldwide are spent on mental disorders [1]. One consequence of this is that in all countries, most people who are mentally ill receive no treatment at all [2;3]. A recent general population survey in the USA, for example, found that 70% of mentally ill people went entirely untreated [4], while a European study showed about three quarters of all people with mental illness went without treatment [5]. The implication is clear: in all countries expenditure on mental health care falls far short of meeting the challenge to provide enough care to all people needing treatment for mental illness. In short, the coverage of care is grossly inadequate: need far outstrips care provision [2;6–10].

Within countries there are also substantial *variations in budgetary inputs*. As discussed in Chapter 8, population level needs for services vary, largely in relation to social deprivation [11;12], because the prevalence of people with severe mental illness and their use of services are far higher in socially deprived areas. By comparison, in many countries financial allocations for mental health care to more and to less socially deprived regions are the same, so penalising the poorer areas from delivering an equivalent quality of care [6].

A related point is the distinction between the *absolute* and the *relative budget* allocations. While the total budgetary 'cake' is usually fixed for mental health services each year, it is possible, by focusing attention in financial discussions only upon changes in proportionate expenditure, to miss opportunities to increase the absolute amount spent. For example, in the period after a major mental health scandal, or just after a new government or minister for health has come into office, there may be a brief opportunity to increase the priority attached to mental health. The converse is that in periods of financial cutbacks, it is vital to ensure that mental health services do not have financial reductions greater than those applied to other areas of healthcare (a form of structural/systemic stigma) [13]. Therefore in allocating funds to local areas for mental health services, several factors need to be kept in mind which can increase mental health service needs:

- Immigrants, refugees and asylum seekers
- Presence of major transport ports or termini bringing unwell people to a local area
- Hostels or shelters for the homeless or for people with severe mental illness
- The concentration of people near to a former large psychiatric hospital
- Specialist institutions for people with complex needs (e.g. social care and nursing homes for disabled people, including older adults; people with learning disabilities; people with addiction disorders) where rates of mental illness can be expected to be high
- Prisons and other types of custodial/detention centre.

What is shared in common at the country/regional level is that *policy inputs* are set which influence each lower level of practice. These higher-level policies can take a number of forms: statutes which have the force of law, official guidance which may be obligatory or discretionary, and codes of practice by the professions which codify reasonable clinical practice.

An illustration of inputs relevant at the country/regional level is the creation and dissemination of *clinical guidelines and protocols*. While these two words are often used as synonyms, in fact the Concise Oxford Dictionary defines a guideline as 'a principle or criterion guiding or directing action', and it defines a protocol as 'the rules, formalities etc. or procedure, group etc.' [14]. In other words protocols give clear instructions on specific clinical interventions, while guidelines offer less specific advice, and allow practitioners to depart from the guidelines if they can justify this on a case-by-case basis. There is now an increasing tendency to align clinical practice with the recommendations contained within such guidelines and protocols. Their aim is to improve clinical outcomes by reducing the variability between an evidence-based (or expert-consensus based) recommendation of best practice and what actually occurs in clinical settings.

Inputs at the local level

Local budgets for mental health services often include both health and social care monies. There may also be contributions from housing departments, from universities, or from education budgets (e.g. for children and adolescent services). In short, the overall financial picture is often complex, and not widely understood. The total resource available for mental health is therefore often more than that from the health ministry alone. Further, in many countries the budget allocations to local areas are made centrally at the national level, and the range of local discretion is rather limited. Nevertheless, the implications of this are that there need to be senior managers in the local service who understand the whole financial picture, and who can convene the various agencies involved in providing mental health care into an effective collaboration, to fully exploit the full range of local discretion that is possible.

At the local level it is important to consider different types of *boundary*. For example, there are boundaries: (i) between different teams within the mental health services; (ii) between health and social care organisations and (iii) between public, for-profit and not-for-profit organisations. At each boundary dysfunctional (poorly managed) relationships can and often do produce inefficiency. In our view the most effective way to manage these multiple boundary issues is to adopt a *whole-system* view to bring together lead personnel from the entire range of stakeholders to agree (usually through service-level agreements or local contracts) the relationships across these boundaries.

For example, in many countries a large part of the mental health budget is spent on the care of long-stay psychiatric inpatients whose clinical condition is largely stable. Should this cost be paid by the health service or by the social-care budget? In Sweden, for example, a law has transferred responsibility and funds for longer-term patients in hospital, who no longer require active medical treatment, from the health to the social service authorities. This measure is designed to be an incentive for social services to move such patients from hospital to cheaper and more appropriate residential care as soon as possible. A similar regulation has been introduced in Italy, where there is the additional implication that families may need to make co-payments for social care, but not for health care costs.

An important input issue that arises at the local level is the balance of expenditure between hospital and community services [15]. In recent years, in most economically developed countries, this shifting balance has been in one direction – from hospital to community [16]. A parallel shift has taken place in moving acute psychiatric in-patient care from large psychiatric institutions to local general hospitals. Each of these changes can be assessed by setting budget targets for where money is spent, and then tracking actual expenditure over time.

Two important points need to be recognised here. Those managing such a process need to ensure that funds follow the patients, otherwise clinical activity shifts rapidly from hospital to community sites, but over two thirds of the budget typically remains at the hospital [17]. Second, during decentralisation there is the ever-present risk that monies will leak out of the mental health system and into other areas of medicine unless the budget holders are extremely astute and guard against such financial predation.

To allow comparison of inputs at the local level we need a common currency of measures. While hospital services traditionally use the total number of available *beds* as the prime indicator of the scale of the input, community services do not, as yet, have even such an over-simplified unit of measurement. It is unlikely that for community services only one indicator will be sufficient to describe such complex systems. Rather we shall need an array of quantitative and qualitative indices [8].

Inputs at the individual level

One of the central themes of this book is that the primary purpose of mental health services at the country/regional and at the local levels is to deliver services to individuals which improve their outcomes. We can therefore see the individual level as a final common pathway for all inputs from the higher levels. We shall describe in this section two main types of input at the individual level: the skills and knowledge of staff (which influence treatment processes), and the delivery of information to individuals and their carers.

Regarding the *skills and knowledge of staff*, it is expertise (or competence) rather than experience or qualifications which is of central importance [18]. This means implementing continuing professional development/continuing medical education, changing focus from practitioner knowledge to skills, and moving from teaching based upon a traditional curriculum to an emphasis upon clinical skills which are evidence-based (see Chapter 11 on clinical processes).

The second main type of individual patient input is *information*. There is an increasing concern about the need to provide information to individuals before obtaining their consent to perform investigations or to provide treatments. In this context we refer to information about diagnosis, course and outcome of the condition, about the types of treatment available, and about the wanted and unwanted effects of these treatments. The reasons for this interest are *legal* (for example, to warn patients about the adverse effects of drugs), *ethical* (it is increasingly becoming routine clinical practice to allow the patient to make informed choices) and *evidential*, since patients who are well informed about treatments are more likely to be satisfied with the service and therefore to adhere to treatment recommendations [19].

Although this need is now widely acknowledged, the practice of conveying information to patients and their families is still usually rather informal. The evidence from general health care suggests that information is most effectively transferred if a stepwise procedure is followed by clinicians:

(1) Ask if the patient wants any information at all.
(2) Make a list of the specific questions the patient wants answered.
(3) Take the questions one at a time and for each one ask what the patient already knows.
(4) Confirm or challenge correct or misinformed statements by the patient.
(5) Offer a short series of statements in answer to each question.
(6) Ask if this is sufficient detail or if the patient wants further elaboration for each point.
(7) Tell the patient that you would like to know if you have been able to answer each question by asking them to summarise what you have said.
(8) Either confirm correct statements by the patient, or rephrase your own presentation of information if the patient has misunderstood or not retained the key points at all.
(9) Repeat this sequence for each of the topics the patient has selected.

How can all these inputs at the individual level be synthesised? In a sense, one of the key tasks of clinicians and practitioners is to interpret the available information inputs (e.g. diagnostic or needs assessments, and clinical guidelines or protocols) *for* each individual, and to translate these into a care plan to be agreed *with* that particular person.

Key points in this chapter

- *Inputs* are those resources which are introduced into the mental health system.
- If the primary purpose of a mental health service is to deliver effective interventions to individuals with mental illness, then inputs are *only* worthwhile if they contribute directly or indirectly towards improved outcomes for individuals.
- Visible inputs include: budgets, staff, buildings, facilities and equipment.
- Invisible inputs include: working relationships, policies and regulations, public stigma and media representations of mental illness.
- A common shortcoming in practice is not offering enough information (an input) to service-users and to family members.
- In all countries, resource inputs mean that no more than a quarter of people with mental illness receive treatment.

REFERENCES

1. World Health Organisation. *Mental Health Atlas 2005*. Geneva: World Health Organisation; 2005.
2. Thornicroft G. Most people with mental illness are not treated. *Lancet* 2007; **370** (9590): 807–808.

3. Wang PS, Guilar-Gaxiola S, Alonso J, *et al*. Use of mental health services for anxiety, mood and substance disorders in 17 countries in the WHO world mental health surveys. *Lancet* 2007; **370**(9590): 841–850.

4. Kessler RC, Demler O, Frank RG, *et al*. Prevalence and treatment of mental disorders, 1990 to 2003. *N. Engl. J. Med.* 2005; **352**(24): 2515–2523.

5. Alonso J, Angermeyer MC, Bernert S, *et al*. Use of mental health services in Europe: results from the European Study of the Epidemiology of Mental Disorders (ESEMeD) project. *Acta Psychiatr. Scand. Suppl.* 2004; (420): 47–54.

6. Patel V, Araya R, Chatterjee S, *et al*. Treatment and prevention of mental disorders in low-income and middle-income countries. *Lancet* 2007; **370**(9591): 991–1005.

7. Patel V, Farooq S and Thara R. What is the best approach to treating schizophrenia in developing countries? *PLoS Med.* 2007; **4**(6): e159.

8. Chisholm D, Flisher A, Lund C, *et al*. Scale up services for mental disorders: a call for action. *Lancet* 2007; **370**(9594): 1241–1252.

9. Prince M, Patel V, Saxena S, *et al*. No health without mental health. *Lancet* 2007; **370** (9590): 859–877.

10. Saxena S, Thornicroft G, Knapp M and Whiteford H. Resources for mental health: scarcity, inequity, and inefficiency. *Lancet* 2007; **370**(9590): 878–889.

11. Tello JE, Jones J, Bonizzato P, *et al*. A census-based socio-economic status (SES) index as a tool to examine the relationship between mental health services use and deprivation. *Soc. Sci. Med.* 2005; **61**(10): 2096–2105.

12. Tello JE, Mazzi M, Tansella M, *et al*. Does socioeconomic status affect the use of community-based psychiatric services? A South Verona case register study. *Acta Psychiatr. Scand.* 2005; **112**(3): 215–223.

13. Schomerus G, Matschinger H and Angermeyer MC. Preferences of the public regarding cutbacks in expenditure for patient care: are there indications of discrimination against those with mental disorders? *Soc. Psychiatry Psychiatr. Epidemiol.* 2006; **41**(5): 369–377.

14. Soanes C and Stevenson A. *Concise Oxford English Dictionary*, 11th edn. Oxford: Oxford University Press; 2003.

15. Thornicroft G and Bebbington P. Deinstitutionalisation – from hospital closure to service development. *Br. J. Psychiatry* 1989; **155**: 739–753.

16. Olson RP. *Mental Health Systems Compared: Great Britain, Norway, Canada and the United States*. Springfield, IL: Charles C. Thomas; 2006.

17. Saxena S, Thornicroft G, Knapp M and Whiteford H. Resources for mental health: scarcity, inequity, and inefficiency. *Lancet* 2007; **370**(9590): 878–889.

18. Roth A and Fonagy P. *What Works for Whom? A Critical Review of Psychotherapy Research*, 2nd edn. New York: Guildford Press; 2004.

19. Lasalvia A, Bonetto C, Tansella M, Stefani B and Ruggeri M. Does staff-patient agreement on needs for care predict a better mental health outcome? A 4-year follow-up in a community service. *Psychol. Med.* 2007;1–12.

11

The time dimension: the process phase

Defining the process phase

The Concise Oxford Dictionary defines process as 'a course of action or proceeding, especially a series of stages in manufacture or some other operation' or as 'the progress or course of something.' [1]

We define as *process* 'those activities which take place in the delivery of mental health care'.

In relation to the theme of this book, the *process phase* therefore refers to a wide range of activities (clinical and non-clinical) which occur in the mental health system (see Table 11.1).

These processes include direct interventions for people with mental illness (such as admissions to hospital, prescriptions of medications or the provision of psychological treatment) as well as non-clinical processes (such as administrative activities). Although our primary emphasis is upon outcomes (see Chapter 12), processes are important because they affect outcomes in important ways. For example, a staff decision of whether to admit a person to hospital or not, or a decision to take or not to take medication as prescribed, by a person with mental illness (two types of clinical process), may have serious implications for that person's treatment outcome. There may also be complex interactions between different processes. For example, increased individual satisfaction with services (perhaps because of better information provision) can improve consequent treatment adherence.

Process at the country/regional level

The many processes taking place within the whole mental health care system are largely invisible unless they are systematically described in ways that allow comparisons between places or across time. Such descriptions of processes at the national level can have several important uses, for example to describe trends

Table 11.1 Overview of the matrix model, with examples of key issues in the process phase

Place Dimension	Time Dimension		
	(A) Input phase	**(B) Process phase**	**(C) Outcome phase**
(1) Country/ regional level	1A	1B • Performance/activity indicators (e.g. admission rates, compulsory treatment rates)	1C
(2) Local level	2A	2B • Service contacts and patterns of service use • Pathways to care and continuity • Targeting of services to special groups	2C
(3) Individual level	3A	3B • Content of therapeutic interventions (both psychological, social and pharmacological) • Continuity of clinical staff • Frequency of appointments	3C

in service delivery and use, such as an investigation which suggests that providing home treatment teams to offer crisis care at home can reduce psychiatric hospital admission rates by up to 20% [2]. Further uses of processes measures include to:

• Allow international comparisons
• Identify areas of relative over- and under-provision
• Establish whether national targets are being met by using indicators.

In fact, specific measures have been used to assess healthcare processes for over half a century [3]. For example, since 1954 the 'management by results' approach has been advocated, using targets as tools for health policy development and implementation. This depends upon the consistent availability of epidemiological data. This approach was central to the targets set by the WHO in 1998 in its Health for All declaration [4]. Such targets are one mechanism available to national, regional or local governments [5–7], and can identify targets that are transparent, controllable and adaptable [8; 9], but there is currently no consensus on indicators that should be used routinely at any of these levels [5].

The World Health Organisation (WHO) Project Atlas was launched in 2000 to collect, compile and disseminate information about mental health resources in different countries, and much of this data concerns processes [10]. Information regarding 16 themes is presented for each of the 192 WHO Member States, for example on staffing levels per 100 000 population, and on the presence or absence of specific mental health policies, programmes and laws. The Atlas was updated in 2005 and the validity of the data improved by incorporating sources other than government officials in the countries concerned [11]. Data at these two time points allowed trends to be analysed and the main findings for the 2001–2005 period were that there were no substantial changes in the resources available for mental health care; regional imbalances in resource availability remained largely stable; and modest increases occurred in community rather than hospital service, the number of mental health professionals and in the number of countries with mental health policies, legislation and essential drug lists [11;12].

A more detailed international set of service comparators are collected in the World Health Organisation Assessment Instrument for Mental Health Systems (WHO-AIMS) [13], again largely consisting of process measures. This consists of 155 indicators covering six domains: policy and legislative framework; mental health services; mental health in primary health care; human resources; public education and links with other sectors; monitoring and research. Together these domains are intended to form a relatively complete picture of a national mental health system, and country-specific reports using this system have been produced for 18 countries.

Process at the local level

We shall discuss here examples of the processes of mental health care which are relevant at the local level: (i) case registers and other local information systems; (ii) the pathways of individuals to and through care, and how far services offer continuity and (iii) the targeting of specialist services to more disabled groups of individuals.

Compared with the country/regional level, process data gathered at the local level using *case registers* can be more detailed. By co-ordinating data from different local sources it is possible to obtain cumulative information for identified individuals. The recent development of electronic patient record systems now means that routine local data systems can now be used as the basis for administrative and monitoring purposes. For example, in Denmark a national psychiatric case register exists which builds a longitudinal record of patterns of hospital care for individual patients, and which is used to link census and other socio-demographic data, both for aetiological epidemiological research (to identify risk factor for psychiatric disorders) [14;15] and for the evaluation of mental health service utilisation [16;17].

Some of the types of data which can be collected using this system at the local level are shown in Table 11.2, most of which monitor local mental health care processes.

Such process measures can be used for the descriptive use of *monitoring* care over time, which may be valuable for administrative purposes. *Evaluating* care is a more complex exercise, and although process variables are often used *as if*

Table 11.2 Definitions of variables which may be used to describe the process of care at the local level

- **Annual treated incidence**: Total number of patients who had a first-ever contact with a psychiatric service during the specified year
- **Annual treated prevalence**: Total number of patients who had a contact with psychiatric services during the specified year
- **One-day treated prevalence**: All patients in contact with psychiatric service on census day, together with patients with a current episode of care (i.e. those who had a psychiatric contact both before and after the census day, with less than 91 days between contacts)
- **Long-term patients on one day**: All patients not continuously hospitalised during the previous year (i.e. not long-stay), who, on census day had been in continuous contact with one or more psychiatric services during the previous 365 days or longer, with less than 91 days between each contact
- **In-patient prevalence**: Total number of patients who spent at least one day in hospital in the specified year
- **First-ever admissions**: Total number of first-ever hospital psychiatric admissions in the specified year
- **Re-admissions**: Total number of hospital psychiatric re-admissions in the specified year
- **Total admissions**: Total number of hospital psychiatric admissions with a date of admission in the specified year[a]
- **Mean number of beds occupied per day**: Mean number of beds occupied in each day
- **Mean length of stay**: Mean duration of stay for all admissions starting in the specified year
- **Admission rates for patients in contact with the services**: In-patients prevalence divided by total treated prevalence, expressed as a percentage
- **In-patient care priority index for a specific diagnostic group**: Total number of days spent in hospital per patient in the specified year for a particular diagnostic group as a ratio of the same figure for patients with all diagnoses
- **Day-hospital prevalence**: Total number of patients who had at least one contact (or visit) at day hospitals or at rehabilitation groups of community mental health centre in specified year
- **Mean day-hospital contacts**: Mean number of day-hospital contacts per day-patient in the specified year
- **Day-hospital care priority index**: Total number of days spent in day hospital for specific diagnostic groups in the specified year as a ratio of the same quantity for patients with all diagnoses
- **Out-patient and casual contacts prevalence**: Total number of patients who had at least one out-patient contact at hospital, community psychiatric clinics (including contacts made with psychiatrist in GP surgeries – for UK only), general hospital liaison and accident and emergency departments in the specified year[b]

Table 11.2 (cont.)

- **Mean out-patient and casual contacts**: Mean number of out-patient and casual contacts per patient treated at this level of care in the specified year
- **Out-patients priority index for specific diagnostic groups**: Total number of out-patients and casual contacts per patients in the year for a particular diagnostic group as a ratio of the same figure for patients with all diagnoses
- **Home visits and community contacts prevalence**: Total number of patients who had at least one visit made to their home or to homes of their friends or relatives, or visits to patients temporarily with other agencies, or visits to premises of voluntary organisations or to social services premises, by psychiatrists, nurses, psychologist and other psychiatric staff in the specified year[b]
- **Mean home visits and community contacts**: Mean number of home visits and community contacts per patient treated at this level of care in the specified year
- **Home visits priority index for specific diagnostic groups**: Total number of home visits and community contacts per patient in the specified year for a particular diagnostic group as a ratio of the same figure for patients with all diagnoses

[a] If a patient was admitted more than once in the specified year, each admission is included in the figure for total admissions.
[b] Only direct face-to-face contacts are included. Any contacts made by telephone are excluded from the counts.
Source: [18]

Table 11.3 Definitions of the severely mentally ill

(1) **National Institute for Mental Health (1987)**
    (i) *Diagnosis* of non-organic psychosis or personality disorder
    (ii) *Duration*, operationalised as a two-year history of mental illness or two years or more of treatment.
    (iii) *Disability*, operationalised as including at least three of:
        (a) Vulnerability to stress
        (b) Disability that prevents self-sufficiency and causes dependency
        (c) Limited ability to obtain needed assistance
        (d) Social behaviour demanding intervention by mental health system or courts
        (e) Impaired activities of daily living and basic needs
        (f) Impaired social functioning
        (g) Limited and impaired performance in employment
        (h) Limited and impaired performance in non-work (e.g. leisure and homemaking).
(2) **Ruggeri *et al.* (2000)** [20]
    (i) *Duration*: operationalised as a two-year or more history of contact with mental health services
    (ii) *Disability*: Global Assessment of Functioning scale score of 50 or less

they were meaningful alone, in fact for evaluation purposes they are incomplete without reference to their associated inputs and outcomes.

A further important set of local process issues are individuals' *pathways* to and through mental health services. The term pathway describes the routes taken by individuals in making a first contact with health services (see *accessibility* in Chapter 4), and the subsequent sequence of events within an episode of care (see *continuity* in Chapter 4). These sequences are highly dependent upon the availability of services locally, and also upon historical patterns of referral and treatment between agencies. An analysis of individuals' pathways can reveal key local system weaknesses, such as points at which referrals fail to connect, or areas of wasteful overlap, where several agencies provide similar services.

The third issue which we shall discuss in relation to the process of care at the local level is *targeting*. Although this is somewhat controversial [19], there is a broad consensus that the people who should receive priority for specialist mental health services are those who are most disabled, to whom services should be provided in relation to need. The concept of severe mental illness has been developed as a form of shorthand to describe particular groups of people who are mentally ill who should receive the highest priority for services (Table 11.3). Until recently this concept was used to refer to people with psychotic disorders, but more recent analyses, using case register data in Verona, found that the prevalence of severe mental illness was 1.34/1000 for people with psychotic disorders, and 0.98/1000 for non-psychotic disorders [20]. In other words there were almost as many people with severe mental illness with non-psychotic as with psychotic disorders.

Figure 11.1 shows a scheme to demonstrate the frequency of mental illnesses in the general community and what proportions are detected and treated in countries which have a reasonably well-functioning primary and secondary health care system. Each year over a quarter of the general population have a mental disorder sufficiently severe to interfere with everyday life [21]. In the UK, for example, approximately between a half and two thirds are detected by primary health care practitioners [22], and only about 2% of the whole adult population are referred to specialist mental health care for assessment or treatment (of whom about a quarter are admitted to a psychiatric hospital each year). The main point is that of all people with mental disorders, only about 10% are seen by specialist staff in economically developed nations. So which 10% should be targeted by specialist services?

If a specialist mental health service decides to target its care to the people who are most disabled by mental illness, how can it check that this is actually happening? One method is to undertake a survey or census of patients treated in local primary care and/or specialist (secondary) care services, assessing their diagnosis, duration of treatment and degree of disability to identify the severely mentally ill group. These results can be compared with estimates of, for

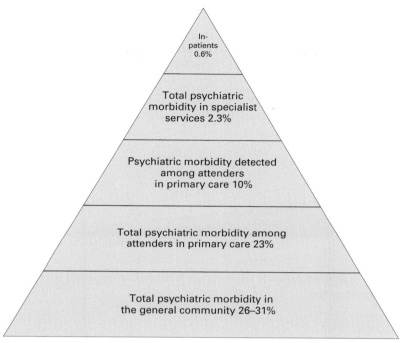

Figure 11.1 Goldberg and Huxley model of psychiatric morbidity.

example, the prevalence of psychotic disorder in the general population (see Chapter 2) to understand what proportion of these people are not receiving any treatment or care at all [23]. The result of such a survey may show a picture similar to that in Figure 11.2 where people with severe mental illness are equally likely to receive no care (A), or to be seen in primary (B) or secondary care (C) – in other words this is a poorly targeted service.

By comparison, a well-targeted service (in more economically developed countries) is one in which most people with severe mental illness are seen by specialist practitioners, and where most people with mild to moderately severe disabling conditions are treated in primary care settings, for example using collaborative care [24;25], as shown in Figure 11.3. Further, in well-targeted systems, individuals who do not have a diagnosed mental illness, after assessment, do not continue to receive treatment, although a recent large survey in the USA found that half of people receiving psychiatric treatment in primary or secondary care settings in fact did not have a diagnosable psychiatric condition (see Chapter 2) [21].

Targeting is necessary, but not sufficient. A crucial further factor is whether the *capacity* of the secondary (specialist) service is large enough to provide cost-effective care to all the cases that fulfil the criteria for severe mental illness.

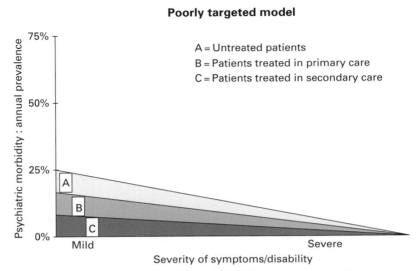

Figure 11.2 Relationship between degree of disability and treatment setting in a poorly targeted service.

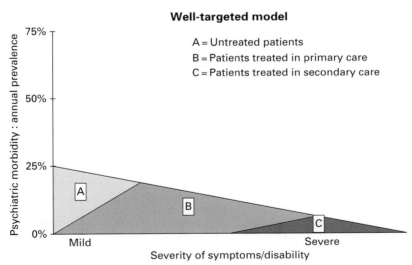

Figure 11.3 Relationship between degree of disability and treatment setting in a well-targeted service.

Process at the individual level

At the individual level, it is striking that the question of what processes happen in meetings between mental health staff and individuals in routine clinical consultations (the content of treatment) have been given insufficient attention and are poorly understood [26]. Efforts to move clinician behaviour towards evidence-based practice, for example by following treatment guidelines and protocols, have produced rather modest effects, characteristically about 10% improvements in clinical outcomes [27–29].

The key implications that arise from this are the importance of manualising treatments specific to particular conditions, to identify the active ingredients of complex interventions (such as case management), and to implement on a widespread basis effective means to ensure behaviour change by practitioners to more closely conform with evidence-based guidelines and protocols. One consequence of this approach is that manualised treatments (such as cognitive-behavioural treatment) do specify how often treatment consultation should take place, whereas in traditional out-patient clinics there is no clear evidence on the most effective frequency of contact [30;31].

What is the relationship between local and individual processes? One way to understand this is to see local processes, such as the activities of community mental health teams, as the *vehicles* to deliver services. At the same time the therapeutic activities of practitioners can be seen as processes at the individual level, which may or may not be therapeutic, according to whether these staff provide effective care to people with mental illness, in other words, if they offer the active ingredients of treatment. A well-functioning mental health service will be coherent in that such active treatments (including methods of optimising the therapeutic relationship, increasing trust and effective communication skills) are *available* from well-trained staff (individual process), and are actually *delivered* to targeted groups of people with mental illness via carefully organised services (local process).

Key points in this chapter

- We define processes as 'those activities which take place in the delivery of mental health care'.
- Processes include direct interventions (such as admissions to hospital, prescriptions of medications, or the provision of psychological treatment) as well as non-clinical (such as administrative) activities.
- Country/regional level processes include such activity indicators as admission rates.
- Local-level process measures include care pathways.

- Individual-level processes refer, for example, to continuity of clinical staff, or frequency of appointments.
- Many mental health service indicators are process measures, as they are more easily available than outcomes, and are sometimes misleadingly used 'as if' they are outcomes.
- The World Health Organisation regularly compiles international comparisons of mental health indicators, most of which are process measures.
- Important aspects of a mental health system are how far it seeks to target services to particular groups of people with mental illness (e.g. those with the greatest levels of disability) and how far it succeeds in doing this.
- Many service innovations (such as community mental health teams) are complex treatment-delivery processes, and to improve outcomes they need to deliver effective treatments.

REFERENCES

1. Soanes C and Stevenson A. *Concise Oxford English Dictionary*, 11th edn. Oxford: Oxford University Press; 2003.
2. Glover G, Arts G and Babu KS. Crisis resolution/home treatment teams and psychiatric admission rates in England. *Br. J. Psychiatry* 2006; **189**(5): 441–445.
3. Van Herten LM and Gunning-Schepers LJ. Targets as a tool in health policy. Part I: Lessons learned. *Health Policy* 2000; **53**(1): 1–11.
4. Van Herten LM and Van de Water HP. New global Health for All targets. *BMJ* 1999; **319**(7211): 700–703.
5. Mainz J, Krog BR, Bjornshave B and Bartels P. Nationwide continuous quality improvement using clinical indicators: the Danish National Indicator Project. *Int. J. Qual. Health Care* 2004; **16** (Suppl 1): i45-i50.
6. Shield T, Campbell S, Rogers A, *et al.* Quality indicators for primary care mental health services. *Qual. Saf. Health Care* 2003; **12**(2): 100–106.
7. Coop CF. Balancing the balanced scorecard for a New Zealand mental health service. *Aust. Health Rev.* 2006; **30**(2): 174–180.
8. Van Herten LM and Gunning-Shepers LJ. Targets as a tool in health policy. Part II: Guidelines for application. *Health Policy* 2000; **53**(1): 13–23.
9. Thornicroft G and Tansella M. *The Mental Health Matrix: A Manual to Improve Services*. Cambridge: Cambridge University Press; 1999.
10. World Health Organisation. *Mental Health Atlas 2001*. Geneva: World Health Organisation; 2001.
11. World Health Organisation. *Mental Health Atlas 2005*. Geneva: World Health Organisation; 2005.
12. Saxena S, Sharan P, Garrido M and Saraceno B. World Health Organization's Mental Health Atlas 2005: implications for policy development. *World Psychiatry* 2006; **5**(3): 179–184.

13. World Health Organisation. *World Health Organisation Assessment Instrument for Mental Health Systems (WHO-AIMS)*. Geneva: World Health Organisation; 2005.
14. Dalton SO, Mellemkjaer L, Thomassen L, Mortensen PB and Johansen C. Risk for cancer in a cohort of patients hospitalized for schizophrenia in Denmark, 1969–1993. *Schizophr. Res.* 2005; **75**(2–3): 315–324.
15. Li J, Laursen TM, Precht DH, Olsen J and Mortensen PB. Hospitalization for mental illness among parents after the death of a child. *N. Engl. J. Med.* 2005; **352**(12): 1190–1196.
16. Munk-Olsen T, Laursen TM, Videbech P, Rosenberg R and Mortensen PB. Electroconvulsive therapy: predictors and trends in utilization from 1976 to 2000. *J. ECT* 2006; **22**(2): 127–132.
17. Erlangsen A, Mortensen PB, Vach W and Jeune B. Psychiatric hospitalisation and suicide among the very old in Denmark: population-based register study. *Br. J. Psychiatry* 2005; **187**: 43–48.
18. Gater R, Amaddeo F, Tansella M, Jackson G and Goldberg D. A comparison of community-based care for schizophrenia in south Verona and south Manchester. *Br. J. Psychiatry* 1995; **166**(3): 344–352.
19. Andrews G. Efficacy, effectiveness and efficiency in mental health service delivery. *Aust. N. Z. J. Psychiatry* 1999; **33**(3): 316–322.
20. Ruggeri M, Leese M, Thornicroft G, Bisoffi G and Tansella M. Definition and prevalence of severe and persistent mental illness. *Br. J. Psychiatry* 2000; **177**: 149–155.
21. Kessler RC, Demler O, Frank RG, *et al.* Prevalence and treatment of mental disorders, 1990 to 2003. *N. Engl. J. Med.* 2005; **352**(24): 2515–2523.
22. Goldberg D and Huxley P. *Common Mental Disorders: A Bio-Social Model*. London: Routledge; 1992.
23. Perala J, Suvisaari J, Saarni SI, *et al.* Lifetime prevalence of psychotic and bipolar I disorders in a general population. *Arch. Gen. Psychiatry* 2007; **64**(1): 19–28.
24. Gilbody S, Bower P, Fletcher J, Richards D and Sutton AJ. Collaborative care for depression: a cumulative meta-analysis and review of longer-term outcomes. *Arch. Intern. Med.* 2006; **166**(21): 2314–2321.
25. Von Korff M and Goldberg D. Improving outcomes in depression. The whole process of care needs to be enhanced. *BMJ* 2001;(323): 948–949.
26. Thornicroft G. Testing and retesting assertive community treatment. *Psychiatr. Serv.* 2000; **51**(6): 703.
27. Gilbody S, Whitty P, Grimshaw J and Thomas R. Educational and organizational interventions to improve the management of depression in primary care: a systematic review. *JAMA* 2003; **289**(23): 3145–3151.
28. Gilbody SM, Whitty PM, Grimshaw JM and Thomas RE. Improving the detection and management of depression in primary care. *Qual. Saf. Health Care* 2003; **12**(2): 149–155.
29. Grimshaw J, Eccles M and Tetroe J. Implementing clinical guidelines: current evidence and future implications. *J. Contin. Educ. Health Prof.* 2004; **24** (Suppl 1): S31–S37.
30. Thornicroft G and Tansella M. The components of a modern mental health service: a pragmatic balance of community and hospital care. *Br. J. Psychiatry* 2004; **185**: 283–290.
31. Becker T. Out-patient psychiatric services. In Thornicroft G and Szmukler G (Eds.). *Textbook of Community Psychiatry*. Oxford: Oxford University Press; 2001: 277–282.

12

The time dimension: the outcome phase

Defining the outcome phase

Outcome is defined in the Concise Oxford Dictionary as 'a result, a visible effect'. In this sense an outcome is the final step of the sequence: inputs, processes and outcomes. In healthcare, outcomes are generally considered to be changes in functioning, in morbidity or in mortality [1]. As with inputs and processes, outcomes can be considered at the three levels of the matrix model (see Tables 12.1 and 12.2).

Process measures, or even input measures, are often used *as if* they are outcomes. This is not only because of confused definitions, but also because our ability to define and measure outcomes in mental health care is not yet well developed. Nevertheless, in the final section of this chapter we shall summarise recent advances in outcome assessment.

Outcomes at the country/regional level

In epidemiology, the classic outcome measures at the population level are mortality and morbidity. Recent work assessing the national and international impact of mental disorders has used a set of standard 'currencies', namely disability adjusted life years (DALY), which refers both to mortality and years lived with disability (YLD) [2;3]. Table 12.3 shows that when disability outcomes are considered separately from mortality, for young adults worldwide, 7 of the top 20 causes of disability are psychiatric disorders, and the conditions causing greatest disability are unipolar depressive disorder, alcohol-use disorders and schizophrenia. Indeed globally 33% of the years lived with disability (YLD) are due to neuropsychiatric disorders, and unipolar depressive disorders alone lead to 12.15% of years lived with disability. Adding in the effects of mortality, then neuropsychiatric conditions account for 13% of disability adjusted life years (DALYs) [4]. These two measures (DALY

Table 12.1 Overview of the matrix model, with examples of key issues in the outcome phase

Place Dimension	Time Dimension		
	(A) Input Phase	**(B) Process Phase**	**(C) Outcome Phase**
(1) Country/ Regional Level	1A	1B	1C • Overall suicide rates • Homelessness rates • Imprisonment rates • Disability adjusted life years • Years lived with disability
(2) Local Level	2A	2B	2C • Suicide rates for people with mental illness • Employment rates • Physical morbidity rates
(3) Individual Level	3A	3B	3C • Symptom severity • Impact on care-givers • Satisfaction with services • Quality of life • Disability • Met and unmet needs

Table 12.2 Outcome measures for use in clinical practice

	Place Dimension		
Outcome measure	**Country level**	**Local level**	**Individual level**
Employment status	✓	✓	✓✓
Physical morbidity	✓	✓	✓
Suicide and self-harm	✓✓	✓	✓✓
Homelessness		✓	✓✓
Standardised mortality ratios	✓	✓	
Symptom severity		✓	✓✓
Impact on care givers		✓	✓
Satisfaction with services		✓	✓✓
Quality of life		✓	✓
Disability		✓	✓✓
Met and unmet needs for care		✓	✓

Key: ✓ =suitable for use as an outcome, ✓✓ =commonly used as an outcome

Table 12.3 Leading causes of years of life lived with disability (YLDs), for 15–44 year olds, estimates for 2000 [2]

Both sexes, 15–44 year olds		% total
1	Unipolar depressive disorders	16.4
2	Alcohol use disorders	5.5
3	Schizophrenia	4.9
4	Iron-deficiency anaemia	4.9
5	Bipolar affective disorders	4.7
6	Hearing loss, adult onset	3.8
7	HIV/AIDS	2.8
8	Chronic obstructive pulmonary disease	2.4
9	Osteoarthritis	2.3
10	Road traffic accidents	2.3
11	Panic disorder	2.2
12	Obstructed labour	2.1
13	Chlamydia	2.0
14	Falls	1.9
15	Asthma	1.9
16	Drug use disorders	1.8
17	Abortion	1.6
18	Migraine	1.6
19	Obsessive-compulsive disorder	1.4
20	Maternal sepsis	1.2

and YLD) are therefore potentially useful outcome measures at the national/ regional level.

Directly in relation to the national/regional level, a frequently used outcome measure is suicide rate (which often also includes self-inflicted injury). This is a particularly useful outcome measure because official data are available for up to the last 25 years for many countries worldwide, in the WHO Mortality Database [5] at www.who.int/healthinfo/morttables/en/index.html. The completeness, accuracy and reliability of these data of course may vary between countries. By comparison the national/regional outcome measure of *home-lessness* among people with mental illness is highly meaningful, but much less available than suicide rate information [6;7].

The fact that such meaningful outcome variables are usually missing is a reflection of the fact that mental health services are seen to be a relatively low priority in many countries. Although, as we have discussed in Chapter 2, mental illnesses make a major contribution to total mortality and morbidity at the national level, it is common for governments to see mental illnesses as of lesser importance than most other conditions. This, combined with a tendency to use process variables that are relatively easy to collect (rather than those which are important), such as hospital admission rates, means that we are usually poorly informed at the country/regional level about how far mental health services achieve their goals.

Outcomes at the local level

At the local level there is a stark distinction between those outcome measures which could theoretically be used, and those which are actually used. As Table 12.2 shows, it is very uncommon for outcomes to be defined, collected and used at the local level. What are the reasons for this? One is that the clinical professions most often involved in research (psychiatrists and psychologists), who usually create and test outcome measures, have a training that focuses on the individual level, whereas those professions routinely involved in running local services (managers and financial officers) much less often have expertise in research. Second, local systems of care are highly complex. If we have difficulty understanding the active ingredients in complex individual level interventions (such as case management), then these difficulties are even greater in trying to know which of the many influences from a whole system of care are effective in promoting the recovery of people with mental illness. There is a further paradox here: community mental health services are deliberately organised on a local level, but they are not assessed at the local level. By comparison, local-level outcome data are routinely collected in many surgical services, for example for deaths and complications rates between different hospitals. For surgery, having a simple dichotomous outcome measure (alive or dead at follow-up) considerably simplifies this procedure. In mental health care there is, as yet, no consensus on what constitutes recovery from an episode of mental illness [8;9]. Finally, there are usually no clear incentives or sanctions to develop and use local-level outcome measures.

There is a recent trend in many countries to publish league tables of indicators on various aspects of health service performance, for example post-operative infection rates, to allow health 'consumers' to have access to information to support their treatment choices. Some of these indicators are local-level outcomes, such as service satisfaction as rated by service-users. We expect that this will be a growing trend and that consumer demand for information about competing health care providers will fuel the development of local-level performance indicators, some of which will be outcome measures [10;11]. One example is how far the needs of groups of service-users in local services are met or unmet, assessed by aggregating assessments of individual needs [12].

Outcomes at the individual level

In our view the primary purpose of mental health services is to optimise outcomes for individuals with mental illness [cell 3C in the matrix model]. In this case, the contributions of all activities in the other cells in the matrix *only* matter if they directly or indirectly contribute to improved individual outcomes. At present, at all three levels, most attention is paid to inputs into mental health care, and to a lesser extent to some processes. We suggest, using this approach, that a balanced overview is necessary which gives clear attention to inputs and processes in so far as they contribute to better outcomes.

How does this way of thinking help us? One example is to use this way of thinking when considering new service developments. In this case if a new community mental health centre is being considered or planned, then key staff involved in this development can ask themselves the challenging question: will this new centre (combining new local resource inputs and local processes) contribute to improved outcomes for individuals with mental illness? In other words we propose a relentless focus upon: (i) if staff and services improve service-user outcomes, (ii) if they do then how do they achieve this and (iii) do these gains offer good value for money?

We shall consider next individual outcome measures (see Table 12.2). These days outcomes assessment is more comprehensive than in previous decades as new measures, beyond symptom severity, have been developed and validated, and particularly because service-users have demanded that a wider range of service impacts be assessed as meaningful to them [13;14]. A further important dimension for assessing treatment outcomes is the impact of carers and family members, and several scales have been carefully developed to measure these implications of care [15;16]. As health care is increasingly seen as the provision of competing products within a marketplace, so there has been more importance attached in recent years to service-users' satisfaction with services, with the associated development of scales to measure this [17;18].

Quality of life ratings have also become more commonly used during the last decade, and several instruments have been made which assess this or the related idea of subjective wellbeing [14;19–21]. Similarly several assessments have been created to measure needs, including both met and unmet needs, and this concept is used to refer to the sometimes differing views of what service-users, family members and staff identify as needs in each particular case [12]. Indeed recent research strongly suggests that the ratings of unmet needs by service-users may be most informative, for example in being closely associated with quality of life [22;23].

Psychometric properties of outcome measures

While an airline pilot would not consider flying a plane without an altimeter that was carefully calibrated, it is still relatively common in mental health care to use measures that have not been properly standardised. Briefly, such standardisation most often refers to the validity and to the reliability of a scale [1].

A research instrument should first of all actually measure what it is intended to measure – it should be valid. There are several ways to assess the validity of a scale:

(1) *Face validity*, which is the subjective judgement made by the user of the instrument about whether the individual items cover the appropriate range of problems relevant to the measure as a whole.
(2) *Content validity* describes whether a scale uses information from all the items it contains.
(3) More widely, the opinions of experts in the field may be taken about a new measure to provide an estimate of *consensual validity*.
(4) *Criterion-related validity* is high when a new measure produces the same result as another instrument whose validity has already been established, where the latter is called the criterion measure.
(5) *Construct validity* addresses the psychological meaning of the test scores.

In addition, a rating scale must give repeatable results for the same service-user when used under different conditions, that is, it must be *reliable*. There are four widely used methods to assess reliability:

(1) *Inter-rater* reliability refers to how far two or more independent raters agree when using the same measure to rate the same person.
(2) *Test-retest* reliability describes how far the score of a rating scale remains constant when used by the same rater with the same person at two or more points in time.
(3) *Parallel form* reliability is measured by having two different, but equivalent, versions of the rating scale, for example with items in a different order.
(4) *Split-half* reliability is a measure of the association between the different halves of the same test, for example between odd and even numbered items.

The main point is that wherever possible it is important to use rating scales, both for clinical as well as research purposes, which have details of their psychometric properties published, and which are known to be at least moderately strong.

Methods for assessing outcomes

What types of evidence can be used to inform decision-making in mental health? A widely used scheme, shown in Table 12.4, arranges five types of evidence in a hierarchy.

Often in mental health care we need to know if complex interventions (such as combined pharmacological and psychological treatments) work or not. How can we assess if such complex treatments (new or old) are effective and cost-effective? One clear framework is that developed by the Medical Research Council in the UK, shown in Figure 12.1 [25]. This proposes five sequential stages: pre-clinical (clarifying the theoretical basis of an intervention); modelling

Table 12.4 Hierarchy of evidence

(1) Evidence from at least one good systematic review
(2) Evidence from at least one good randomised controlled trial (RCT)
(3) Evidence from at least one controlled study without randomisation
(4) Evidence from at least one well-designed observational study
(5) Expert opinion, including the opinion of service-users and carers

Source: [24]

(writing a manual to clearly describe the intervention); exploratory trial (a relatively small study to see if the new intervention appears to be effective); definitive trial (a large study, usually a randomised controlled trial) to definitively establish if the intervention is effective and cost-effective; and long-term implementation (the putting of the new intervention into widespread routine practice).

Sometimes RCTs are defined either as *efficacy* trials (which assess a new intervention under ideal or experimental conditions) or *effectiveness* trials (which assess how far a new intervention works under ordinary, routine clinical conditions). To inform mental health service decisions, information from effectiveness trials is far more useful [26]. A further important issue in interpreting research evidence for mental health service planning and provision is to understand when associations between variables are causally important. Bradford Hill has described several criteria that are helpful for this purpose, as shown in Table 12.5.

Using outcome measures in routine clinical practice

Is it feasible to use routine outcome measures in routine clinical practice? While it is common for some clinical teams to use outcomes for all patients, it is relatively uncommon for whole mental health systems to use outcomes on a regular basis. An exception is several states in Australia, which have implemented the use of the HoNOS scale on a widespread basis [28;29]. Similarly in South Verona in Italy all patients in contact with specialist mental health care are assessed every six months with standardised outcome assessments [30;31]. How can we know if it is feasible to use particular scales in ordinary clinical practice [32]? Feasibility can be assessed in terms of:

- Brevity (looks short and easy to use)
- Simplicity (no training required, meaning of ratings is clear)
- Relevance (accords with clinical judgement, no jargon)
- Acceptability (to professions, suitable for flexible administration)
- Availability (free, and can be photocopied easily)
- Value (little time needed for data entry, and feedback is clinically useful).

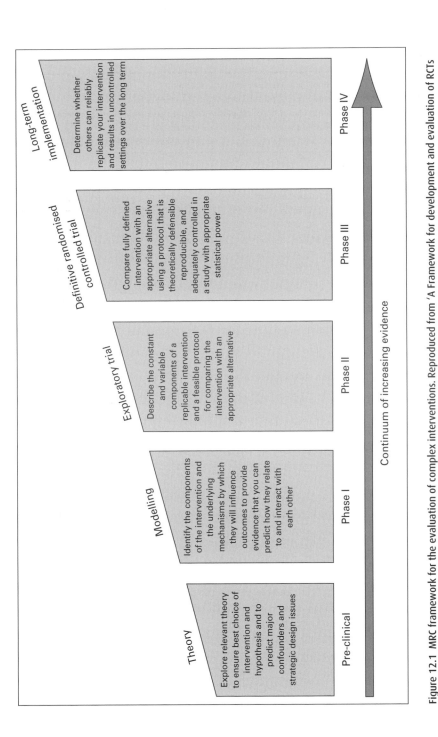

Figure 12.1 MRC framework for the evaluation of complex interventions. Reproduced from 'A Framework for development and evaluation of RCTs for Complex Interventions to Improve Health' issued on 1st April 2000 by MRC. Reproduced with permission.

Table 12.5 Bradford Hill's criteria for causality

- Strength of the association (whether the correlation between two variables is high)
- Consistency (if an association has been 'repeatedly observed')
- Specificity (whether a particular consequence follows *only* from a specific intervention)
- Temporality (if a change in the first variable always occurs before a change in the second variable)
- Biological gradient (is there a dose–response relationship)
- Plausibility (is an association acceptable in the wider context of scientific knowledge)
- Coherence (is the association in line with other relevant research evidence)
- Experimental evidence (is there supportive evidence from intervention trials)

Source: [27]

The central idea of this book is the primary importance of paying attention to the outcomes for individuals with mental illness. For this to be a core part of everyday clinical practice it requires that outcome measurement is an accepted part of mental health care, and that such data are collected for all people treated by services on a regular basis.

Key points in this chapter

- We propose that the primary purpose of mental health services is to improve outcomes for individuals with mental illness.
- It therefore follows that the accurate and routine assessment of outcomes is an essential aspect of care.
- An example of outcomes at the country/regional level is suicide rates.
- At the local level employment rate for people with mental illness may be a relevant outcome measure.
- At the individual level, outcome can be assessed in terms of symptom severity, impact on care-givers, satisfaction with services, quality of life, disability or met and unmet needs
- It is important for clinical and research use to choose measures that have well-established psychometric properties

REFERENCES

1. Tansella M and Thornicroft G (Eds.). *Mental Health Outcome Measures*. London: Royal College of Psychiatrists, Gaskell; 2001.
2. World Health Organisation. World Health Report 2001. *Mental Health: New Understanding, New Hope*. Geneva: World Health Organization; 2001.

3. Murray C and Lopez A. *The Global Burden of Disease, Vol. 1. A Comprehensive Assessment of Mortality and Disability from Diseases, Injuries and Risk Factors in 1990, and Projected to 2020.* Cambridge, MA: Harvard University Press; 1996.

4. World Health Organisation. *Investing in Mental Health.* Geneva: World Health Organisation; 2003.

5. WHO. *WHO Mortality Database.* Geneva: World Health Organisation; 2006.

6. Folsom DP, Hawthorne W, Lindamer L, *et al.* Prevalence and risk factors for homelessness and utilization of mental health services among 10340 patients with serious mental illness in a large public mental health system. *Am. J. Psychiatry* 2005; **162**(2): 370–376.

7. Bhui K, Shanahan L and Harding G. Homelessness and mental illness: a literature review and a qualitative study of perceptions of the adequacy of care. *Int. J. Soc. Psychiatry* 2006; **52**(2): 152–165.

8. Warner R. *Recovery from Schizophrenia: Psychiatry and Political Economy.* Hove: Brunner-Routledge; 2004.

9. Lester H and Gask L. Delivering medical care for patients with serious mental illness or promoting a collaborative model of recovery? *Br. J. Psychiatry* 2006; **188**: 401–402.

10. McEwan KL and Goldner EM. Keeping mental health reform on course: selecting indicators of mental health system performance. *Can. J. Commun. Ment. Health* 2002; **21**(1): 5–16.

11. Dausey DJ, Rosenheck RA and Lehman AF. Pre-admission care as a new mental health performance indicator. *Psychiatr. Serv.* 2002; **53**(11): 1451–1455.

12. Slade M, Thornicroft G, Loftus L, Phelan M and Wykes T. *CAN: The Camberwell Assessment of Need.* London: Gaskell, Royal College of Psychiatrists; 1999.

13. Chamberlin J. User/consumer involvement in mental health service delivery. *Epidemiol. Psichiatr. Soc.* 2005; **14**(1): 10–14.

14. Thornicroft G, Becker T, Knapp M, *et al. International Outcome Measures in Mental Health. Quality of Life, Needs, Service Satisfaction, Costs and Impact on Carers.* London: Gaskell, Royal College of Psychiatrists; 2006.

15. Van Wijngaarden B, Schene AH, Koeter M, *et al.* Caregiving in schizophrenia: development, internal consistency and reliability of the Involvement Evaluation Questionnaire – European Version. EPSILON Study 4. European psychiatric services: inputs linked to outcome domains and needs. *Br. J. Psychiatry Suppl.* 2000;(39): s21-s27.

16. Szmukler GI, Burgess P, Herrman H, *et al.* Caring for relatives with serious mental illness: the development of the Experience of Caregiving Inventory. *Soc. Psychiatry Psychiatr. Epidemiol.* 1996; **31**(3–4): 137–148.

17. Ruggeri M, Dall'Agnola R, Agostini C and Bisoffi G. Acceptability, sensitivity and content validity of the VECS and VSSS in measuring expectations and satisfaction in psychiatric patients and their relatives. *Soc. Psychiatry Psychiatr. Epidemiol.* 1994; **29** (6): 265–276.

18. Ruggeri M, Dall'agnola R, Bisoffi G and Greenfield T. Factor analysis of the Verona Service Satisfaction Scale-82 and development of reduced versions. *Int. J. Meth. Psychiatr. Res.* 1996; **6**(1): 23–38.

19. Lehman AF. Measures of quality of life among persons with severe and persistent mental disorders. *Soc. Psychiatry Psychiatr. Epidemiol.* 1996; **31**(2): 78–88.

20. Meijer CJ, Schene AH and Koeter MWJ. Quality of life in Schizophrenia measured by the MOS SF36 and the Lancashire Quality of Life Profile: a comparison. *Acta Psychiatr. Scand.* 2002; **105**(4): 293.

21. Ware J and Sherbourn C. The MOS, 36 item Short-Form Health Survey (SF-36). I Conceptual framework and item selection. *Med. Care* 1992; **30**: 473–483.

22. Slade M, Leese M, Ruggeri M, *et al.* Does meeting needs improve quality of life? *Psychother. Psychosom.* 2004; **73**(3): 183–189.

23. Lasalvia A, Bonetto C, Malchiodi F, *et al.* Listening to patients' needs to improve their subjective quality of life. *Psychol. Med.* 2005; **35**(11): 1655–1665.

24. Department of Health. *National Service Framework: Mental Health.* London: Department of Health; 1999.

25. Campbell M, Fitzpatrick R, Haines A, *et al.* Framework for design and evaluation of complex interventions to improve health. *BMJ* 2000; **321**(7262): 694–696.

26. Tansella M, Thornicroft G, Barbui C, Cipriani A and Saraceno B. Seven criteria for improving effectiveness trials in psychiatry. *Psychol. Med.* 2006; **36**(5): 711–720.

27. Hill B. The environment and disease: association or causation? *Proc. Royal Soc. Med.* 1965; 295–300.

28. Trauer T. Routine outcome measurement by mental health-care providers. *Lancet* 2003; **361**(9363): 1137.

29. Wing JK, Beevor AS, Curtis RH, *et al.* Health of the Nation Outcome Scales (HoNOS). Research and development. *Br. J. Psychiatry* 1998; **172**: 11–18.

30. Ruggeri M, Leese M, Slade M, *et al.* Demographic, clinical, social and service variables associated with higher needs for care in community psychiatric service patients. The South Verona Outcome Project 8. *Soc. Psychiatry Psychiatr. Epidemiol.* 2004; **39**(1): 60–68.

31. Lasalvia A and Ruggeri M. Multidimensional outcomes in 'real world' mental health services: follow-up findings from the South Verona Project. *Acta Psychiatr. Scand. (Suppl.)* 2007; **116**: 3–77.

32. Slade M, Thornicroft G and Glover G. The feasibility of routine outcome measures in mental health. *Soc. Psychiatry Psychiatr. Epidemiol.* 1999; **34**(5): 243–249.

13

The central role of staff for better mental health care

At the outset we need to distinguish between *primary* and *secondary service goals*. By *primary goals* we mean the treatment and care of people with mental illness. In our view this is the main purpose of the service and should always remain centre stage. By *secondary goals* we mean meeting the needs of staff. We shall argue in this chapter that unless these staff needs are properly met, the quality of service will suffer.

To a much greater extent than most other areas of medicine, mental health services rely almost entirely upon human resources rather than upon techno-logical devices. For example, the clinical interview is still the most valid method to establish the diagnosis. In terms of treatment, it is clear that the therapeutic relationship and the human skills of clinicians are of central importance in influencing how far service-users choose to adhere to treatment recommenda-tions, and so have better outcomes.

There are important implications for this central role of the human factor. Apart from capital (buildings) costs, recurrent expenditure in mental health services is almost entirely needed for the development and maintenance of human resources. Further, the nature of clinical contact with people with mental illness puts demands upon staff that draw upon all their reserves, and which render staff at risk of a depletion of motivation and compassion, the so-called 'burnout syndrome'. Staff are therefore not fixed resources, but are continually subject to deterioration or degradation unless maintained and renewed.

Changing from an institutional to a community perspective

Moving from a mental health system dependent upon hospitals to one which is a balance of hospital and community services implies far more than only a physical relocation of treatment sites. It entails also a fundamental reorienta-tion of perspective. In part this requires new staff attitudes. Table 13.1 shows staff attitudes typical of the two approaches (expressed as distinct for clarity,

Table 13.1 Differences in staff attitudes between institutional and community perspectives

	Institutional Perspective	Community Perspective
Staff Attitudes	• Seeing service-users (usually referred to as patients within institutional settings) within the hospital context • Focus on symptoms and behavioural control • Planned/routine contacts • Guidance from set policies and procedures • Hierarchical decision-making and command structure (often medical model) • Stronger belief in pharmacological treatments • View that service-users with severe symptoms should remain in hospital • Paternalistic attitude that staff are responsible for the behaviour of service-users • View that service-users in hospital are not responsible for their own anti-social behaviour and that these should not be reported to police	• Seeing service-users within the home and family context • Focus on needs of the individual and the family • Flexibility: planned and unplanned contacts • Responses to changing needs of service-users • Emphasis on shared decision-making and negotiation (between staff, and between staff and service-users) • Combining pharmacological, psychological and social interventions • View that symptoms do not necessarily determine the correct care setting for each person • Empowering emphasis on the responsibilities of each service-user along with their choices and consequences • Service-users assumed to be responsible for their behaviour and to undergo due legal process if committing a crime

although in practice, mixed attitudes along these axes are common, and may vary according to the disciplinary background of staff members). Within institutions, hierarchical and traditional structures predominate, with a focus on control, order, routine and the medicalisation of treatment and care. Within the balanced care model there is a refocusing upon individualised care, involving service-users and family members in care decisions, and upon staff of all disciplines having a greater degree of professional autonomy than is common in traditional hospital settings, within the context of multi-disciplinary team work.

Table 13.2 shows key distinctions between the basic professional training receiving by staff in institutional and community settings. While the former typically takes place only in traditional hospital and out-patient sites, the latter will usually consist of training rotations or placements in a much wider range

Table 13.2 Differences in staff training between the institutional and community perspectives

	Institutional Perspective	Community Perspective
Staff Training	• More biological training orientation • Separate training curricula for different practitioners • Training only takes place in hospital and clinic settings • Training on specialist units for different diagnostic groups • Focus on diagnostic formulation	• Eclectic bio-psycho-social orientation • Some shared training element across disciplines • Training takes place in hospital and in community settings • Training is often in teams providing for mixed diagnostic groups (e.g. for a catchment area) • Focus on assessing unmet needs

of clinical settings, including, for example, community mental health teams, residential care, day centres, rehabilitation workshops, and within primary care centres and general hospitals.

Further, therapeutic orientation will vary according to the care setting, as shown in Table 13.3. For example, commonly community-based services will tend to pay greater attention to assessing and treating people with mental illness in their own home, and will assess a wider range of their clinical and social needs. More fundamentally, the community orientation to a large extent seeks to assist people with mental illness in leading their own lives according to their own specific priorities and goals (putting staff in a facilitatory or supportive role), rather than maintaining the paternalistic view that staff are responsible for virtually all aspects of the lives of those whom they treat.

Basic and continuing professional education

In any cycle of changing mental health services, two training challenges are present: (i) how to re-orientate staff who have already completed their basic professional education and (ii) how to change the basic training curricula for future staff. As we have emphasised throughout this book, decisions here can be guided by referring to the relevant ethics, evidence and experience to shape what is done locally. Priorities for training are likely to be highly specific to each time and place. For example, in part of Eastern Europe where there is no established tradition of psychiatric social workers, then creating such practitioners may be a high priority. One example of a framework for training (in this case used in England) is known as 'Shared Capabilities in Mental Health Practice', as shown in Table 13.4 [1], although this particular set of core elements may not be directly applicable to other situations.

Table 13.3 Differences in therapeutic orientation between the institutional and community perspectives

	Institutional Perspective	Community Perspective
Therapeutic Orientation	• Emphasis on symptom relief • Improved facilities and expertise for physical assessment, investigation, procedures and treatment • Seek decision from above in the hierarchy • Focus on control of violent behaviour • Block treatment for groups of individuals • Regulated timetable • Separated short-term treatment and rehabilitation • Culture which tends to avoid risk taking • Commonly clinical and administrative leadership is assumed to be held by medical doctors (which may maintain closer links with other medical specialities)	• Greater focus on service-user empowerment • Risk of less focussed attention on physical health, even to the neglect of this aspect • More autonomy for staff in different disciplines • Sees behaviour more often with specific contexts • More individualised treatment and care • Flexibility in when and where service-users are treated • Integrated therapeutic and social interventions • Culture which will try new approaches to services and to care plans • Leadership can be exercised by any discipline (which may be seen to make mental health services distinct and distant from other medical specialities)

Training guided by evidence: treatment guidelines

We take it as a vital starting point to this discussion that staff should deliver treatments that work and not waste resources in undertaking interventions that are ineffective or even those which are known to be harmful. We therefore suggest that the training of mental health practitioners should be based as far as possible upon an 'evidence-based medicine (EBM)/evidence-based practice (EBP)' approach. The most common method intended to translate evidence into practice is the generation of treatment guidelines, which have the following advantages [2]:

• Implementation of 'best practice' psychiatric treatment
• Education of psychiatrists, other physicians and other mental health professionals
• Provision of information to the people with mental illness and their families
• Improved funding of psychiatric services

Table 13.4 Ten essential shared capabilities in mental health practice [1]

(1) **Working in partnership**. Developing and maintaining constructive working relationships with service-users, carers, families, colleagues, lay people and wider community networks. Working positively with any tensions created by conflicts of interest or aspiration that may arise between the partners in care.

(2) **Respecting diversity**. Working in partnership with service-users, carers, families and colleagues to provide care and interventions that not only make a positive difference, but also do so in ways that respect and value diversity, including age, race, culture, disability, gender, spirituality and sexuality.

(3) **Practising ethically**. Recognising the rights and aspirations of service-users and their families, acknowledging power differentials and minimising them whenever possible. Providing treatment and care that is accountable to service-users and carers within the boundaries prescribed by national (professional), legal and local codes of ethical practice.

(4) **Challenging inequality**. Addressing the causes and consequences of stigma, discrimination, social inequality and exclusion on service-users, carers and mental health services. Creating, developing or maintaining valued social roles for people in the communities they come from.

(5) **Promoting recovery**. Working in partnership to provide care and treatment that enables service-users and carers to tackle mental health problems with hope and optimism and to work towards a valued lifestyle within and beyond the limits of any mental health problem.

(6) **Identifying people's needs and strengths**. Working in partnership to gather information to agree health and social care needs in the context of the preferred lifestyle and aspirations of service-users, their families, carers and friends.

(7) **Providing service-user-centred care**. Negotiating achievable and meaningful goals; primarily from the perspective of service-users and their families. Influencing and seeking the means to achieve these goals and clarifying the responsibilities of the people who will provide any help that is needed, including systematically evaluating outcomes and achievements.

(8) **Making a difference**. Facilitating access to and delivering the best quality, evidence-based, values-based health and social care interventions to meet the needs and aspirations of service-users and their families and carers.

(9) **Promoting safety and positive risk-taking**. Empowering the person to decide the level of risk-they are prepared to take with their health and safety. This includes working with the tension between promoting safety and positive risk-taking, including assessing and dealing with possible risks for service-users, carers, family members and the wider public.

(10) **Personal development and learning**. Keeping up-to-date with changes in practice and participating in life-long learning, personal and professional development for one's self and colleagues through supervision, appraisal and reflective practice.

- Identification of 'gaps' in the research base and promotion of more effective research
- Increased recognition of the scientific basis of the treatment of mental illnesses.

At the same time the use of guidelines needs to be considered also in light of their limitations, namely: (i) lack of implementation; (ii) gaps in research base; (iii) a sometimes overly reductionistic (medical model) approach to medical care; (iv) unknown cross-cultural applicability of interventions; (v) liability concerns when practitioners do or do not follow guidelines and (vi) the feasibility of following guidelines where available resources are very limited, for example in low- and medium-income countries. Nevertheless, for several mental disorders there are now many different guidelines available. One recent survey, for example, identified 27 guidelines from 21 countries for the treatment of people with schizophrenia [3].

Since the content of such guidelines (especially for psycho-social interventions) varies a great deal, how can one decide which guidelines to follow? One approach uses the six Appraisal Guideline Research Evaluation-Europe (AGREE) criteria to assess the quality of guidelines: scope and purpose of the guideline; stakeholder involvement; rigour of development; clarity of presentation; applicability and editorial independence [3]. Interestingly, of all 27 guidelines rated using these criteria, the UK NICE Schizophrenia Guidelines were the most highly rated. Across all the guidelines assessed, the most frequently occurring evidence-based interventions were:

- Anti-psychotic medication
  - First-line and acute-relapse regimes
  - Treatment-resistant cases and use of clozapine
  - Dosage for maintenance therapy after first and after subsequent episodes
  - First-line management of side effects
  - Minimisation of polypharmacy
  - Use of anti-depressants for depressive symptoms.
- Psycho-social interventions
  - Provision of family support
  - Psycho-social interventions
  - Psychological therapy/cognitive-behavioural therapy
  - Systems of vocational rehabilitation
  - Systems of community treatment.

The important issue here is that these effective interventions need to be available to treat people with mental illness – in this illustration people with schizophrenia. Mental health systems vary a great deal, for example, in how many doctors or nurses or social workers are available, or even whether mental health staff are available at all. Therefore it is important that the staff who are available, whatever their professional background, are trained with the necessary skills to deliver these specific evidence-based interventions. In other situations, for example in rural/remote areas, then primary care staff may be the only personnel able to give direct evidence-based care, or it may be more feasible to use tele-medicine techniques may provide the necessary expertise, or self-help methods, such as the use of computerised cognitive-behavioural treatment programmes for depression [4;5].

Implementing guidelines in routine practice

If training is provided in evidence-based skills, will this lead to better routine clinical care? Unfortunately, the evidence suggests: not necessarily. Indeed passive knowledge transfer activities appear to be largely ineffective, although the evidence base on how to implement guidelines is at present weak, especially for economic studies and for research that relates to improved service-user outcomes [6–12]. The active ingredients which appear to be necessary for successfully putting guidelines into practice include:

- Development of a concrete proposal for change
- Analysis of the target setting and group to identify obstacles to change
- Linking interventions to needs, facilitators and obstacles to change, e.g. educational outreach (for prescribing) and reminders
- Development of an implementation plan
- Monitoring progress with implementation.

One use for guidelines is to assess, for a particular clinical service, how far staff routinely provide good clinical practice as defined by a specific set of guidelines, and to identify gaps in the provision of clinical care which need to be rectified, for example by employing additional staff or by training staff to provide additional evidence-based interventions. For example, in a recent survey in Italy, 19 mental health services nationwide rated their care against 103 pre-specified criteria from the NICE guidelines for the treatment of schizophrenia [13;14]. Illustrating the general point that *what cannot be measured cannot be managed*, this set of indicators provided a clear picture of the quality of care given to people with schizophrenia, and showed great variation across Italy, especially in how far treatments were targeted to the illness at onset and if psychological treatments were provided early in the condition (both to people with schizophrenia and to their family members). Such an assessment can provide a valuable baseline to assess in future whether clinical care more often conforms to evidence-based practice (Ruggeri, in preparation).

Apart from staff skills, therapeutic attitudes are also important. We propose a distinction between the specific clinical skills identified by guidelines, and the overall desirable attitudes of staff. Table 13.5 shows both desirable and undesirable characteristics of staff in a balanced mental health service. Indeed staff attitudes may at least be as important as the treatment setting: for example,

Table 13.5 Characteristics of community mental health staff (Mosher and Burti, 1989) [15]

Desirable characteristics

- Strong sense of self: comfort with uncertainty
- Open minded: accepting and non-judgmental
- Patient and non-intrusive
- Practical, problem-solving orientation
- Flexible
- Empathic
- Optimistic and supportive
- Gentle firmness
- Humorous
- Humble
- Thinks contextually

Undesirable characteristics

- The rescue fantasy
- Consistent distortion of information
- Pessimistic outlook
- Exploits clients for own needs
- Over-controlling and needing to do for others
- Suspicious and blaming others

former hospital staff may (re)create a stronger institutional atmosphere in small group homes than in a large psychiatric institution.

Building and maintaining clinical teams

The clinical team can be seen both as a collection of individual practitioners, and as a vehicle for providing care in its own right. The characteristics of a team as a whole include the clinical setting, the style of leadership and the degree of co-ordination with other teams. From our own experience and in the views of international panel of commentators (see Chapter 6) the following factors promote positive team working:

- Clear vision from the team leader of the primary task of the team
- Clarification of roles for each team member
- Specific operational policies, for example about the purpose of the team, appropriate service-user referrals to the team, how transfers from the team are managed and maximum case load
- Active methods to engage service-users and family members in seeking feedback on the team's performance

- Investment in the clinical environment (e.g. buildings and furniture) that shows that value is attached to high-quality treatment settings
- Integration of all the relevant disciplines into single clinical teams, often including nursing, medical, psychological, social work and occupational therapy staff
- Shared clinical records systems
- Clear protocols (e.g. on how service-users can be admitted to and discharged from hospital), which are mutually agreed across the relevant service interface
- Continuing professional development provided for individual staff training needs
- An atmosphere in which staff can challenge each other to improve clinical practice.

A useful scheme is to think of the clinical team in four stages: new team building; major reconstruction; maintenance and minor reconstruction. Figure 13.1 shows the cyclical relationship between the phases of construction and subsequent team maintenance. When creating a new clinical team, an early task is to define the *purpose of the team*.

A further important element is to set the *boundary conditions*. Setting the boundaries of the team will include identifying: (i) the specific goals and aims of the team within the context of the local mental health system as a whole; (ii) the particular service-user groups to be served, for example on the basis of diagnosis or disability; (iii) the intended duration of clinical contact, or episodes of care, which are indicated by clinical considerations and financial constraints; (iv) the limits of staff duties (for example, powers to physically restrain people, to admit to hospital, or to give injectable depot medication); (v) how far the team is intended to substitute for another component of care, for example whether a home treatment team (crisis resolution team) is meant to reduce psychiatric in-patient admissions [16].

Over a period of years, many clinical teams, both in hospital and in community-based settings, will require some degree of support or organisational change, either to a minor or a major degree. This can be precipitated by changes in key staff, such as the team leader/manager, the senior psychiatrist or psychologist. In our experience, clinical teams vary a great deal in how far they are stable over time and how much active attention is required to allow them to provide clinical

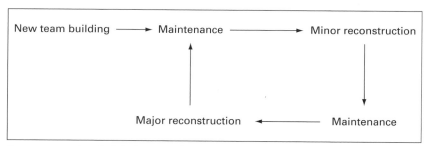

Figure 13.1 Cycles of clinical team building and maintenance.

Table 13.6 Features and causes of staff burnout [15]

Features

- No energy
- No interest in clients
- Clients frustrating, hopeless or untreatable
- Higher absenteeism
- High staff turnover
- Demoralisation

Causes

- Setting too hierarchical: staff not empowered
- Too many externally introduced rules, no local authority and responsibility
- Work group too large or non-cohesive
- Too many clients, feels overwhelmed
- Too little stimulation, repetitive routine work practices

care well. It cannot be assumed that teams will operate effectively, unless attention is paid to the clarity of their role and the quality of their management.

To a large extent clinical teams are successful if their staff members are enabled to maintain their clinical effectiveness and to avoid low morale and burnout. Burnout is a term which has come to be widely used and recognised as the consequence of prolonged and severe role strain. It is a dysfunctional psychological state that is most common among people working in settings characterised by a great deal of personal interaction, under conditions of chronic stress and tension. These conditions are frequently found in clinical teams, especially those with the features shown in Table 13.6. There are a number of techniques which can be used to prevent or reverse burnout, including: frequent teaching and training sessions; regular staff meetings for inter-personal problem solving; routine case conferences to discuss difficult cases and regular staff supervision [15].

In summary, the clinical team, and its staff members, is the critical bridge between the inputs we identified in Chapter 10 (in so far as it is able to organise, manage and deliver the therapeutic processes that we discussed in Chapter 11), intended to achieve the better clinical outcomes for individual service-users, as illustrated in Chapter 12.

Key points in this chapter

- For mental health services, the *primary goal is* the treatment and care of people with mental illness.
- Meeting the needs of staff is a *secondary goal*, nevertheless unless these needs are properly met, the quality of service will suffer.

- To a much greater extent than most other areas of medicine, mental health services rely almost entirely upon human resources rather than upon technological devices.
- Moving services from institutions to the community requires both a physical relocation of treatment sites, and a fundamental re-orientation of staff attitudes.
- Staff training increasingly needs to ensure the acquisition of evidence-based clinical skills, particularly guided by clinical protocols and guidelines.
- Just as hospital buildings need regular maintenance, clinical teams are sustained by careful, regular maintenance activities.

REFERENCES

1. Hope R. *The Ten Essential Shared Capabilities: A Framework for the Whole Mental Health Workforce.* London: Department of Health; 2004.
2. McIntyre JS. Usefulness and limitations of treatment guidelines in psychiatry. *World Psychiatry* 2002; **1**(3): 186–189.
3. Gaebel W, Weinmann S, Sartorius N, Rutz W and McIntyre JS. Schizophrenia practice guidelines: international survey and comparison. *Br. J. Psychiatry* 2005; **187**: 248–255.
4. Proudfoot J, Ryden C, Everitt B, *et al.* Clinical efficacy of computerised cognitive-behavioural therapy for anxiety and depression in primary care: randomised controlled trial. *Br. J. Psychiatry* 2004; **185**: 46–54.
5. Kaltenthaler E, Brazier J, De NE, *et al.* Computerised cognitive behaviour therapy for depression and anxiety update: a systematic review and economic evaluation. *Health Technol. Assess.* 2006; **10**(33): iii, xi–iii,168.
6. Grol R and Grimshaw J. Evidence-based implementation of evidence-based medicine. *Jt. Comm. J. Qual. Improv.* 1999; **25**(10): 503–513.
7. Grol R and Grimshaw J. From best evidence to best practice: effective implementation of change in patients' care. *Lancet* 2003; **362**(9391): 1225–1230.
8. Grimshaw JM, Shirran L, Thomas R, *et al.* Changing provider behavior: an overview of systematic reviews of interventions. *Med. Care* 2001; **39**(8 Suppl 2): II2–45.
9. Gilbody S, Whitty P, Grimshaw J and Thomas R. Educational and organizational interventions to improve the management of depression in primary care: a systematic review. *JAMA* 2003; **289**(23): 3145–3151.
10. Grimshaw J, Eccles M and Tetroe J. Implementing clinical guidelines: current evidence and future implications. *J. Contin. Educ. Health Prof.* 2004; 24 Suppl **1**: S31-S37.
11. Grimshaw JM, Thomas RE, MacLennan G, *et al.* Effectiveness and efficiency of guideline dissemination and implementation strategies. *Health Technol. Assess.* 2004; **8**(6): iii–72.
12. Vale L, Thomas R, MacLennan G and Grimshaw J. Systematic review of economic evaluations and cost analyses of guideline implementation strategies. *Eur. J. Health Econ.* **2007**; 8(2): 111–121.

13. NICE. *Schizophrenia: Full National Clinical Guideline on Core Interventions in Primary and Secondary Care.* London: Royal College of Psychiatrists and British Psychological Society; 2003.

14. Pilling S and Price K. Developing and implementing clinical guidelines: lessons from the NICE schizophrenia guideline. *Epidemiol. Psichiatr. Soc.* 2006; **15**(2): 109–116.

15. Mosher LR and Burti L. *Community Mental Health – Principles and Practice.* New York: W.W. Norton & Co.; 1989.

16. Glover G, Arts G and Babu KS. Crisis resolution/home treatment teams and psychiatric admission rates in England. *Br. J. Psychiatry* 2006; **189**: 441–445.

14

Informed actions for better mental health care

An ambitiously realistic vision for mental health care

In this book we aim to support you in your role, perhaps planning or providing or using mental health services, by providing an overall framework (the matrix model) and by offering a wide range of ideas based upon the best that is currently available in relation to ethics, evidence and experience. What is our longer-term ambition for better mental health care? In a sense our vision is one that provides remedies for the many shortcomings that have been described previously in this book. Here in this concluding chapter we describe a vision for better mental health care that is both ambitious and realistic.

Our proposals start with the recognition (described in Chapter 2) that the difference between the number of people who have mental illnesses and the number who are treated in any way is truly enormous [1]. This 'treatment gap' means that even in the best-resourced countries, about a third of people with the most severely disabling conditions such as schizophrenia, and over two-thirds of people with more common mental disorders, such as anxiety and depression, receive no treatment at all [2]. These findings have wide-ranging implications [3]. They mean that most countries simply do not have the capacity, at present, to respond to the full scale of the challenge to offer treatment and care for people with mental illnesses. As we saw in Chapter 2, even in the richest countries, specialist mental health care treats only up to 3% of the whole adult population each year. The greater number of others who have some form of mental illness, if they are to find help, need to look elsewhere. On the other hand, in some countries, as for example the USA, 10% of the general population are not unwell and yet do receive psychiatric treatment, mainly medication [4]. This paradox is probably due to the insufficient ability of mental health services to be made available to all those in need, and to the imperative of drug companies to optimise their sales performance.

In recent years it has been common to describe the primary/secondary/ tertiary care model (see Chapter 5) and to propose that the extra 'missing' capacity needs to be provided in primary care. The rationale is that all conditions should first be assessed and diagnosed in primary care, acting as a filter or triage stage, and that only the more severe cases, or those not responding to treatment in primary care, should be referred on to mental health specialists. Indeed the balanced care model (that we describe in Chapter 8) is consistent with this received wisdom. On one hand, this approach seems reasonable and the evidence supports the view that common mental disorders are highly prevalent in primary care settings. On the other hand, however, we need to be cautious and not to accept uncritically a service model whose utility has not been systematically evaluated, especially in low-resource settings [5]. More practically orientated research is needed, and meanwhile we need to be cautious in importing models that do not fit local circumstances.

The vast range of different types of health services across the world mean that no one model could possibly apply to all locations. Rather we now need to develop a portfolio of options that draw on a blend of: individual self-management, family-provided care, treatment by whatever health and social support resources are available locally (for example indigenous practitioners, staff and members of church or other faith communities), voluntary associations, non-governmental organisations, with teaching, consultancy and direct clinical care from primary and secondary (specialist) health care (where they exist in any numbers).

Understanding barriers to change

To enact such a vision means eroding, quickly or slowly, a chain of resistant barriers that have often prevented meaningful improvement in mental health care across the globe. The key barriers have been identified as shown in Table 14.1 [6].

It is reasonable to see beneath these surface features of neglect, the signs of an underlying structural discrimination against people with mental illness. In short, the lack of real interest in investing in better health care in most countries shows that, in practice, people with mental illnesses are treated as if they have a lower value than others. One example of such a differential is that non-discrimination laws, in countries where they exist, are usually drafted and implemented in relation to disability from physical rather than mental disorders [7].

Unifying the mental health sector and advocating for resources

The self-advocacy and lobbying power of people with mental illness is currently weak in most countries. Indeed, one of the central paradoxes is that while up to three quarters of adults know someone directly who has been affected by a mental illness, we act as if nobody knows anything [8;9]. One consequence is

Table 14.1 Key barriers and challenges to better mental health care

Barriers	Challenges to overcoming barriers
(1) Insufficient funding for mental health services	<ul><li>Inconsistent and unclear advocacy</li><li>Perception that mental health indicators are weak</li><li>People with mental disorders are not a powerful lobby</li><li>Lack of general public interest in mental health</li><li>Social stigma</li><li>Incorrect belief that care is not cost effective</li></ul>
(2) Mental health resources centralised in and near big cities and in large institutions	<ul><li>Historical reliance on mental hospitals</li><li>Fragmentation of mental health responsibilities between different government departments</li><li>Differences between central and provincial government priorities</li><li>Vested interests of staff in continuing large hospitals</li><li>Political risks associated with trade union protests</li><li>Need for transitional funding to move to community-based care</li></ul>
(3) Complexities of integrating mental health care effectively in primary care services	<ul><li>Primary care workers already overburdened</li><li>Lack of training, supervision and ongoing specialist support</li><li>Lack of continuous supply of relevant medications in primary care</li></ul>
(4) Low numbers and limited types of health workers trained and supervised in mental health care	<ul><li>Poor working conditions in public mental health services</li><li>Lack of incentives for staff to work in rural areas</li><li>Professional establishment opposes expanded role for non-specialists in mental health workforce</li><li>Medical students and psychiatrists trained only in mental hospitals</li><li>Inadequate training of general health workforce</li><li>Mental health specialists spend more time providing care rather than training and supervising others</li><li>Lack of infrastructure to enable community-based supervision</li></ul>

Table 14.1 (cont.)

Barriers	Challenges to overcoming barriers
(5) Mental health leaders often deficient in public-health skills and experience	• Those who rise to leadership positions often only trained in clinical management of individuals, not population level needs • Public health training does not include mental health • Lack of training courses in public mental health • Mental health clinical leaders overburdened by clinical and management responsibilities and private practice
(6) Fragmentation between mental health advocacy groups	• Conceptual and practical differences between consumers and mental health staff, especially about diagnoses and treatments • Divisions between consumer and family member groups • Politicians therefore find it easy to ignore an incoherent message

Adapted from Saraceno *et al.* 2007 [6] with permission.

that those in the mental health field who do have resources at their disposal should selectively provide financial and human support to service-user/consumer groups, at a respectful distance, so that these groups can develop, flourish, identify their own priorities and decide how they can exert pressure to achieve their goals. This can be as simple as making direct financial grants to self-help groups, or providing office space and meeting rooms.

But there is an even more important over-riding priority – for the mental health sector to be better organised and to speak with one voice [6]. When it comes to campaigning for fundamental issues, a practical approach is for local and national agencies to set aside their differences and to find a common cause. This will often mean establishing a single co-ordinating group at the country/regional level, sometimes called a forum, peak body, alliance or consortium. What they have in common is a recognition that what they can achieve together, in political terms, is greater than their impact as separate organisations. Core issues likely to unite such coalitions include: large-scale campaigns against stigma [10]; assessing and implementing the recovery model [11]; achieving parity in funding entitlements [12]; the application of laws against disability discrimination against people with mental illness;

Table 14.2 Interactions between mental disorders and other health conditions

---

Mental disorders can affect the rate of other health conditions

- Mental disorders are associated with risk factors for smoking, reduced activity, poor diet, obesity and hypertension
- Depression has biological effects related to cardiac function, inflammation, clotting, cancer and HIV progression

Some health conditions affect the risk for mental disorders

- Infections (e.g., cerebral malaria, HIV, tuberculosis); cerebro-vascular diseases; diabetes; alcohol and substance use can increase the risk for symptoms of mental illnesses including: cognitive impairment; behaviour disturbance; mood disorders; delusions and hallucinations
- Many chronic diseases create a psychological burden, which arises from factors such as the acute trauma of the diagnosis; the difficulty of living with the illness; the long-term threat of decline and shortened life expectancy; necessary lifestyle changes; complicated therapeutic regimens; aversive symptoms such as pain and stigma, which can lead to guilt, loss of social support, or breakdown of key relationships

Comorbid mental disorders can affect treatment and outcome for physical disorders

- Mental disorders can delay help-seeking, reduce the likelihood of detection and diagnosis, or both
- The extent and the quality of general medical health care received by people with mental disorders tends to be worse
- The evidence for this inequity is especially strong for those with psychoses, dementia and substance misuse
- Mental disorders, cognitive impairment and substance- and alcohol-use disorders adversely affect adherence to treatment of physical disorders

---

Adapted from Prince *et al.* 2007 [17] with permission.

advocating for new mental health laws; greater investment in mental health research leading to better treatments and the recognition of international human rights conventions in practice [13–16]. The lesson from physical health care, such as cancer or HIV treatment, is that such unity can drive up investment in research, training and clinical care. We need more critical evaluation of mental health practice (at the individual level), and of mental health systems of care (especially at the local level). Mental health professionals need to explain more persuasively to service-users the rationale and advantages of evidence-based practice. We therefore envisage a continuing interaction between knowledge stemming from clinical experience and knowledge from scientific evidence, each informing the other in turn.

Beyond the argument for greater direct investment in mental health care is a parallel case that mental illnesses act as barriers to impede the proper treatment of major physical illnesses, as shown in Table 14.2 [17]. There is therefore both a case to argue for greater capacity, effectively to directly treat mental illnesses, and to focus on how they impair the prevention, recognition and treatment of concurrent physical disorders. In practice what shall we do to address this second challenge? We need to provide better access to physical health care for people with mental illness, and to decrease stigmatising attitudes among medical staff [18–20].

Setting targets to measure progress

There is a management saying that what cannot be measured cannot be improved, and in our view clear indicators can be powerful tools to drive towards better mental health care. Internationally, the Millennium Development Goals have set an overall framework for global health improvement, but these do not explicitly address mental disorder [21]. Targets need to be transparent, controllable and adaptable [22], and amenable to measurement at the individual, local or national level [23;24]. There is currently no consensus on which mental health indicators should be used routinely at any of these levels [25], but recently a set of primary and secondary measures, suitable for use at the country/regional and at the local levels has been proposed [26], as shown in Table 14.3.

We suggest that you consider using specific and measurable indicators, both to describe your current mental health services, and to use them in setting targets, so that you can assess at a later period if key components, and key aspects of your system as a whole, have changed, and if they have, whether they have improved or deteriorated.

Better mental health care informed by ethics, evidence and experience

We wish to end by returning to the central proposition of this book: that creating better mental health care means drawing upon the best ethical, evidential and experiential information available to you. The latter two types of information in these three domains will continue to change, so it will be important for you to search for the most current updates when planning and implementing service improvements.

In terms of the wider ethical context, is mental illness the strongest remaining social taboo [27]? Certainly the ways in which many people with mental illness are left in social [28] and material poverty [29] suggest that our societies have long constructed and tolerated forms of 'structural violence' against people with mental illness [30–35].

By using clearer reference to ethical guidelines, one way to counteract stigma and discrimination is to give a far greater practical emphasis to the proper

Table 14.3 Primary and secondary indicators to measure better mental health care [26]. Reproduced with permission from Elsevier, copyright 2007.

	Proposed Indicators	Existing Indicators*	Sources of data
Core Indicators			
Ensure that national and regional health plans pay sufficient attention to mental health	1: Presence of official policy, programmes, or plans for mental health, either including or accompanied by a policy on child and adolescent mental health	Atlas, AIMS (1.1.1, 1.2.1)	National government
Invest more in mental health care	2: Specified budget for mental health as a proportion of total health budget	Atlas, AIMS (1.5.1)	National government
Increase trained staff to provide mental health care	3: Mental health and related professionals per 100 000 population	AIMS (4.1.1)	National government and professional bodies
Make basic pharmacological treatments available in primary care	4: Proportion of primary health-care clinics in which a physician or an equivalent health worker is available, and at least one psychotropic medicine of each therapeutic category (antipsychotic, antidepressant, mood stabiliser, anxiolytic, and antiepileptic) is available in the facility or in a nearby pharmacy all year long	AIMS (3.1.7)	National government
Increase the treatment coverage for people with schizophrenia	5: People treated each year for schizophrenia as a proportion of the total estimated annual prevalence of schizophrenia	AIMS (2.2.4.2, 2.4.4.2, 2.6.5.2)	National government and statistical or academic organisations
Secondary indicators			
Balance expenditure in hospital and community services	6: Proportion of total mental health expenditure spent on community-based services, including primary and general health-care services	AIMS (1.5.2)	National government
Provide adequate basic training in mental health	7: Proportion of the aggregate total training time in basic medical and nursing training degree courses devoted to mental health	AIMS (3.1.1, 3.2.1)	National government and professional bodies
Distribute staff equitably between urban and rural areas	8: Proportion of psychiatrists nationally who work in mental health facilities that are based in or near the largest cities	AIMS (4.1.7)	National government
Ensure least restrictive practice	9: Involuntary admissions as a proportion of all annual admissions	AIMS (2.4.5, 2.6.6)	National government
Protect the human rights of people with mental disorder	10: Presence of a national body that monitors and protects the human rights of people with mental disorders, and issues reports at least every year	AIMS (1.4.1)	National government, professional bodies, and civil-society groups
Reduce the suicide rate	11: Deaths by suicide and self-inflicted injury rate	WHO Mortality database	National government and statistical organisations

* Atlas = WHO Mental Health Atlas, AIMS = WHO Assessment Instrument for Mental Health Systems, Figures in parentheses are AIMS indicator numbers.

observation of human rights in every aspect of mental health care. This means sharpening our sights upon injustice as experienced by people with mental illness [36–39]. People with mental illnesses in many countries are treated in ways which prevent them from exercising some of their basic human rights. Although many legally binding international conventions and declarations apply to disabled people in general, they are at present not often enough applied in practice to people with mental health-related disabilities.

The primary source of international human rights within the United Nations (UN) is the Universal Declaration of Human Rights (UDHR), which refers to civil, political, economic, social and cultural rights. Countries which have ratified the International Covenant on Civil and Political Rights (ICCPR) and the International Covenant on Economic, Social and Cultural Rights (ICESCR) are then obliged under international law to guarantee to every person on their territory, without discrimination, all the rights enshrined in both [40–44].

More specifically in relation to mental illness, the UN Principles for the Protection of Persons with Mental Illness and for the Improvement of Mental Health Care were adopted in 1991, and elaborate the basic rights and freedoms of people with mental illness that must be secured if states are to be in full compliance with the ICESCR. The 'The Right to Mental Health' is stated in Article 12, which provides the right of everyone to the enjoyment of the highest attainable standard of physical and mental health, and identifies some of the measures states should take 'to achieve the full realisation of this right'. They provide criteria for the determination of mental illness, protection of confidentiality, standards of care, the rights of people in mental health facilities and the provision of resources. Mental Illness Principle 1 lays down the basic foundation upon which states' obligations towards people with mental illness are built: that 'all persons with a mental illness, or who are being treated as such persons, shall be treated with humanity and respect for the inherent dignity of the human person', and 'shall have the right to exercise all civil, political, economic, social and cultural rights as recognised in the Universal Declaration of Human Rights, the International Covenant on Economic, Social and Cultural Rights, the International Covenant on Civil and Political Rights and in other relevant instruments'. It also provides that 'all persons have the right to the best available mental health care' [31].

In terms of the treatment interventions offered by practitioners, the research evidence is best embodied in clinical treatment guidelines and protocols [45–47]. Nevertheless although these have been produced in many versions, relatively little is understood about the factors which promote their update and use [48;49]. This is also because not enough research has been dedicated so far to evaluate both how to successfully implement such initiatives, and their impact on outcomes.

An integrating approach that is likely to become increasingly influential in the future is the concept of *care pathways*, which means a sequence of clinical events designed to produce a specific outcome most efficiently (for example, all aspects of a hip replacement). Most definitions of clinical pathways include three specific components: (i) the types of interventions that should be provided; (ii) the timeline and sequence of these interventions and (iii) clarity about who does what. This latter element can be very useful to give written information to service-users/consumers and family members about what they can expect to happen during an episode of treatment, so that they are well enough informed to advocate for themselves if any aspect of care is not provided on time [50–53].

Care pathways are 'both a tool and a concept that embed guidelines, protocols and locally agreed, evidence-based, patient-centred, best practice, into everyday use for the individual patient' [54]. Clinical pathway development and use is more common in other areas of health care than in mental health. The limited evidence on factors which promote their implementation gives findings similar to those for guidelines and protocols, namely to maximise clinical engagement as an essential ingredient.

Finally, we reaffirm the central importance of learning from experience – primarily the experience of people with mental illness and their family members. Our central contention in this book is that the primary aim of mental health care is to achieve better outcomes for individuals with mental illness. As the intended beneficiaries, therefore, people with mental illness need to have a central say in what services are planned, how they are provided, how their impact is assessed: in short – in every aspect of care [55;56]. If there is one defining characteristic that we wish to see embodied in the future, it is that service-users are actually included as full partners in directly contributing to better mental health care.

Key points in this chapter

- Planners need to consider how to provide service coverage for the full range of people with mental disorders within the local population.
- In situations where primary care cannot treat most people with common mental disorders, then more locally specific solutions are needed, for example a blend of: individual self-management; family-provided care; treatment by whatever health and social supports are available locally (for example, indigenous practitioners), voluntary associations and non-governmental organisations.
- Six key barriers to change need to be recognised and challenged: (i) insufficient funding for mental health services; (ii) mental health resources centralised in and near big cities and in large institutions; (iii) complexities of integrating mental health care effectively in primary care services; (iv) low numbers and limited types of health workers trained

and supervised in mental health care; (v) mental health leaders often deficient in public health skills and experience; (vi) fragmentation between mental health advocacy groups.

- To reduce fragmentation, a single co-ordinating group can be established at the country/regional level, speaking with one voice about mental health priorities.
- Mental illnesses also act as barriers to impede the proper treatment of major physical illnesses and so services also need to address these particular barriers.
- If it is accepted that what cannot be measured cannot be improved, then quantified indicators can be powerful tools to measure progress towards better mental health care.
- Many people with mental illness are left in social and material poverty, so one way to counteract stigma and discrimination is to give a greater practical emphasis to the proper observation of human rights in every aspect of mental health care.
- In future we expect that research evidence will be practically embodied in treatment guidelines, protocols and clinical pathways, one advantage of which is to empower service-users/consumers and family members with the information to know what to demand from services.
- We end with the two central propositions of this book: (i) that creating better mental health care means drawing upon the best ethical, evidential and experiential information available to you and (ii) that the primary aim of mental health care is to achieve better outcomes for individuals with mental illness
- These propositions imply that in future, service-users are actually included as full partners in directly contributing to better mental health care

REFERENCES

1. Kohn R, Saxena S, Levav I and Saraceno B. The treatment gap in mental health care. *Bull. World Health Organ.* 2004; **82**(11): 858–866.
2. Wang PS, Aguilar-Gaxiola S, Alonso J, *et al.* Use of mental health services for anxiety, mood, and substance disorders in 17 countries in the WHO world mental health surveys. *Lancet* 2007; **370**(9590): 841–850.
3. Patel V, Saraceno B and Kleinman A. Beyond evidence: the moral case for international mental health. *Am. J. Psychiatry* 2006; **163**(8): 1312–1315.
4. Kessler RC, Demler O, Frank RG, *et al.* Prevalence and treatment of mental disorders, 1990 to 2003. *N. Engl. J. Med.* 2005; **352**(24): 2515–2523.
5. Cohen A and Gureje O. Making sense of evidence. *Int. Rev. Psychiatry* 2007; **19**(5): 583–591.

6. Saraceno B, Van OM, Batniji R, *et al.* Barriers to improvement of mental health services in low-income and middle-income countries. *Lancet* 2007; **370**(9593): 1164–1174.

7. Bartlett P, Lewis O and Thorold O. *Mental Disability and the European Convention on Human Rights.* Leiden: Martinus Nijhoff; 2006.

8. Crisp A, Gelder MG, Goddard E and Meltzer H. Stigmatization of people with mental illnesses: a follow-up study within the Changing Minds campaign of the Royal College of Psychiatrists. *World Psychiatry* 2005; **4**: 106–113.

9. Hinshaw SP and Cicchetti D. Stigma and mental disorder: conceptions of illness, public attitudes, personal disclosure, and social policy. *Dev. Psychopathol.* 2000; **12** (4): 555–598.

10. Dunion L and Gordon L. Tackling the attitude problem. The achievements to date of Scotland's 'see me' anti-stigma campaign. *Ment. Health Today* 2005; 22–25.

11. Slade M and Hayward M. Recovery, psychosis and psychiatry: research is better than rhetoric. *Acta Psychiatr. Scand.* 2007; **116**(2): 81–83.

12. Druss BG. Mental health parity, access, and quality of care. *Med. Care* 2006; **44**(6): 497–498.

13. Mercer S, Dieppe P, Chambers R and MacDonald R. Equality for people with disabilities in medicine. *BMJ* 2003; **327**(7420): 882–883.

14. Hanson KW. Public opinion and the mental health parity debate: lessons from the survey literature. *Psychiatr. Serv.* 1998; **49**(8): 1059–1066.

15. Thornicroft G and Rose D. Mental health in Europe. *BMJ* 2005; **330**(7492): 613–614.

16. Frank RG, Goldman HH and McGuire TG. Will parity in coverage result in better mental health care? *N. Engl. J. Med.* 2001; **345**(23): 1701–1704.

17. Prince M, Patel V, Saxena S, *et al.* No health without mental health. *Lancet* 2007; **370** (9590): 859–877.

18. Leucht S, Burkard T, Henderson J, Maj M and Sartorius N. Physical illness and schizophrenia: a review of the literature. *Acta Psychiatr. Scand.* 2007; **116**(5): 317–333.

19. Disability Rights Commission. *Equal Treatment: Closing the Gap. A Formal Investigation into Physical Health Inequalities Experienced by People With Learning Disabilities and/or Mental Health Problems.* London: Disability Rights Commission; 2006.

20. Thornicroft G. *Shunned: Discrimination against People with Mental Illness.* Oxford: Oxford University Press; 2006.

21. Sachs JD and McArthur JW. The Millennium Project: a plan for meeting the Millennium Development Goals. *Lancet* 2005; **365**(9456): 347–353.

22. Becker L, Pickett J and Levine R. *Measuring Committment to Health. Global Health Indicators Working Group Report.* Washington DC: Centre for Global Development; 2006.

23. Van Herten LM and Gunning-Schepers LJ. Targets as a tool in health policy. Part I: Lessons learned. *Health Policy* 2000; **53**(1): 1–11.

24. Van Herten LM and Gunning-Shepers LJ. Targets as a tool in health policy. Part II: Guidelines for application. *Health Policy* 2000; **53**(1): 13–23.

25. Desjarlais R, Eisenberg L, Good B and Kleinman A. *World Mental Health. Problems and Priorities in Low Income Countries.* Oxford: Oxford University Press; 1995.

26. Chisholm D, Flisher AJ, Lund C, *et al.* Scale up services for mental disorders: a call for action. *Lancet* 2007; **370**(9594): 1241–1252.

27. Soanes C and Stevenson A. *Concise Oxford English Dictionary*, 11th edn. Oxford: Oxford University Press; 2003.

28. Dear M and Wolch J. *Landscapes of Despair*. Princeton: Princeton University Press; 1992.

29. Estroff S. *Making it Crazy: Ethnography of Psychiatric Clients in an American Community*. Berkeley: University of California Press; 1981.

30. Corrigan PW, Watson AC, Gracia G, *et al.* Newspaper stories as measures of structural stigma. *Psychiatr. Serv.* 2005; **56**(5): 551–556.

31. World Health Organisation. *WHO Resource Book on Mental Health, Human Rights and Legislation*. Geneva: World Health Organisation; 2005.

32. Sayce L and Curran C. Tackling social exclusion across Europe. In Knapp M, McDaid D, Mossialos E and Thornicroft G (Eds.). *Mental Health Policy and Practice Across Europe. The Future Direction of Mental Health Care*. Milton Keynes: Open University Press; 2006.

33. Sartorius N and Schulze H. *Reducing the Stigma of Mental Illness. A Report from a Global Programme of the World Psychiatric Association*. Cambridge: Cambridge University Press; 2005.

34. Porter R. Can the stigma of mental illness be changed? *Lancet* 1998; **352**(9133): 1049–1050.

35. Shorter E. *A History of Psychiatry*. New York: John Wiley & Sons, Inc.; 1997.

36. Amnesty International. *Ethical Codes and Declarations Relevant to the Health Professions*. London: Amnesty International; 2000.

37. Kingdon D, Jones R and Lonnqvist J. Protecting the human rights of people with mental disorder: new recommendations emerging from the Council of Europe. *Br. J. Psychiatry* 2004; **185**: 277–279.

38. Mental Disability Advocacy Centre. *Cage Beds*. Budapest: Mental Disability Advocacy Centre; 2003.

39. Social Exclusion Unit. *Mental Health and Social Exclusion*. London: Office of the Deputy Prime Minister; 2004.

40. United Nations. *Universal Declaration of Human Rights. Adopted and Proclaimed by the UN General Assembly Resolution 217A (III) of 10 December 1948*. New York: United Nations; 1948.

41. United Nations. *International Covenant on Civil and Political Rights. Adopted by the UN General Assembly Resolution 2200A (XXI) of 16 December 1966*. New York: United Nations (http://www.ohchr.org/english/countries/ratification/4.htm); 1966.

42. United Nations. *International Covenant on Economic, Social and Cultural Rights. Adopted by UN General Assembly Resolution 2200A (XXI) of 16 December 1966*. New York: United Nations; 1966.

43. United Nations. *UN Principles for the Protection of Persons with Mental Illness and for the Improvement of Mental Health Care. Adopted by UN General Assembly Resolution 46/119 of 18 February 1992*. New York: United Nations; 1992.

44. United Nations. *Persons with Disabilities. General Comments Number 5 (Eleventh Session 1994). UN Doc E/C 12/1994/13. UN Committee on Economic, Social and Cultural Rights*. New York: United Nations; 1994.

45. Bero LA, Grilli R, Grimshaw JM, *et al.* Closing the gap between research and practice: an overview of systematic reviews of interventions to promote the implementation of research findings. The Cochrane Effective Practice and Organization of Care Review Group. *BMJ* 1998; **317**(7156): 465–468.

46. Woolf SH, Grol R, Hutchinson A, Eccles M and Grimshaw J. Clinical guidelines: potential benefits, limitations, and harms of clinical guidelines. *BMJ* 1999; **318** (7182): 527–530.

47. Grol R and Grimshaw J. From best evidence to best practice: effective implementation of change in patients' care. *Lancet* 2003; **362**(9391): 1225–1230.

48. Vale L, Thomas R, MacLennan G and Grimshaw J. Systematic review of economic evaluations and cost analyses of guideline implementation strategies. *Eur. J. Health Econ.* 2007; **8**(2): 111–121.

49. Tugwell P, Robinson V, Grimshaw J and Santesso N. Systematic reviews and knowledge translation. *Bull. World Health Organ.* 2006; **84**(8): 643–651.

50. Evans-Lacko S, Jarrett M, McCrone P and Thornicroft G. Clinical pathways in psychiatry. In submission 2008.

51. Emmerson B, Frost A, Fawcett L, *et al.* Do clinical pathways really improve clinical performance in mental health settings? *Australas Psychiatry* 2006; **14**(4): 395–398.

52. Campbell H, Hotchkiss R, Bradshaw N and Porteous M. Integrated care pathways. *BMJ* 1998; **316**(7125): 133–137.

53. Dy SM, Garg P, Nyberg D, *et al.* Critical pathway effectiveness: assessing the impact of patient, hospital care, and pathway characteristics using qualitative comparative analysis. *Health Serv. Res.* 2005; **40**(2): 499–516.

54. Whittle C. Introduction to ICPs (Integrated Care Pathways). http://www.library. nhs.uk/pathways/ViewResource.aspx?resID=259106&tabID=290&catID=12584. London: National Health Service Protocols and Care Pathways Specialist Library; 2007.

55. Chamberlin J. User/consumer involvement in mental health service delivery. *Epidemiol. Psichiatr. Soc.* 2005; **14**(1): 10–14.

56. Rose D. *Users' Voices, The Perspectives of Mental Health Service Users on Community and Hospital Care.* London: The Sainsbury Centre; 2001.

Index